Praise for *Childhood Disrupted*

"A truly important gift of understanding—illuminates the heartbreaking costs of childhood trauma and, like good medicine, offers the promising science of healing and prevention."

—Jack Kornfield, PhD, author of *A Path with Heart*

"This groundbreaking book connects the dots between early life trauma and the physical and mental suffering so many live with as adults. Nakazawa fully engages us with fascinating, clearly written science and moving stories from her own and others' struggles with life-changing illness. A blend of fresh insight into the impact of trauma and invaluable guidance in turning toward healing!"

—Tara Brach, PhD, author of *Radical Acceptance* and *True Refuge*

"A courageous, compassionate, and rigorous every-person's guide through the common roots and enduring impact of childhood trauma in each of our lives. Artfully leads the reader to take practical steps . . . to heal the legacy of trauma in our personal and collective lives."

—Christina Bethell, PhD, MBH, MPH, professor of child health,
Johns Hopkins Bloomberg School of Public Health

"Masterfully captures the complexity of how early life adversity imprints on our biology and stalks our health into adulthood. Practical advice for remaining unbroken in a challenging world."

—Margaret M. McCarthy, PhD, professor and chair,
Department of Pharmacology, University of Maryland School of Medicine

"Eye-opening and inspiring . . . a paradigm-shifting road map for understanding how early stress is linked to later illness and . . . how to begin healing at any age. Will help readers and especially women better understand the biology of stress, and jump-start important new conversations about our health and well-being!"

—DeLisa Fairweather, PhD,
director of cardiovascular translational research, Mayo Clinic

"Every few years a book comes along that changes the way we view ourselves, our society, and our place in the world. This is such a book. Compulsively readable and deeply moving."

—Shannon Brownlee, MS, author of
Overtreated: Why Too Much Medicine is Making Us Sicker and Poorer and
senior vice president of the Lown Institute

"A must-have book for every person facing mental or physical health challenges and their loved ones—and an inspiring read for every health-care professional."

—Gerard E. Mullin MD, associate professor of medicine at
Johns Hopkins School of Medicine and author of *The Gut Balance Revolution*

"Nakazawa writes compassionately for readers struggling to make sense of what happened during their childhoods and how their health may be affected . . . [An] engaging work of scientific translation."

—*Health Affairs*

CHILDHOOD DISRUPTED

HOW YOUR BIOGRAPHY BECOMES YOUR BIOLOGY, AND HOW YOU CAN HEAL

Donna Jackson Nakazawa

ATRIA PAPERBACK

New York   London   Toronto   Sydney   New Delhi

Note to Readers

This publication contains the opinions and ideas of its author. It is intended to provide helpful and informative material on the subjects addressed in the publication. It is sold with the understanding that the author and publisher are not engaged in rendering medical, health, or any kind of personal professional services in the book. The reader should consult his or her medical, health, or other competent professional before adopting any of the suggestions in this book or drawing inferences from it.

The author and publisher specifically disclaim all responsibility for any liability, loss or risk, personal or otherwise, which is incurred as a consequence, directly or indirectly, of the use and application of any of the contents of this book.

Names and identifying details of some of the people portrayed in this book have been changed, and some people portrayed are composites.

ATRIA PAPERBACK
An Imprint of Simon & Schuster, Inc.
1230 Avenue of the Americas
New York, NY 10020

First Atria paperback edition July 2016

ATRIA PAPERBACK and colophon are trademarks of Simon & Schuster, Inc.

For information about special discounts for bulk purchases, please contact Simon & Schuster Special Sales at 1-866-506-1949 or business@simonandschuster.com.

The Simon & Schuster Speakers Bureau can bring authors to your live event. For more information or to book an event, contact the Simon & Schuster Speakers Bureau at 1-866-248-3049 or visit our website at www.simonspeakers.com.

Designed by Kyoko Watanabe

Manufactured in the United States of America

20 19

Library of Congress Cataloging-in-Publication Data is Nakazawa, Donna Jackson.
   Childhood disrupted : how your biography becomes your biology, and how you can heal / Donna Jackson Nakazawa.
      pages cm
      Includes bibliographical references and index.
   1. Psychic trauma in children. 2. Adult child abuse victims—Mental health. 3. Post-traumatic stress disorder. 4. Parent and child. I. Title.
   RJ506.P66N35 2015
   618.92'8521—dc23
                              2015009059

ISBN 978-1-4767-4835-1
ISBN 978-1-4767-4836-8 (pbk)
ISBN 978-1-4767-4837-5 (ebook)

For Christian, for Claire

CONTENTS

INTRODUCTION   xiii

TAKE THE ADVERSE CHILDHOOD EXPERIENCES (ACE) SURVEY   xxi

PART I

How It Is We Become Who We Are

CHAPTER ONE: Every Adult Was Once a Child   3

The Philosophical Physicians   10

Time Does Not Heal All Wounds   13

The Body Remembers—and Will Tell Its Tale   17

The New Theory of Everything   24

Even "Mild" Childhood Adversity Matters   25

CHAPTER TWO: Different Adversities Lead to Similar Health Problems   28

How Your Biography Becomes Your Biology   29

Why Stress Is More Damaging to a Child   31

Medical Adverse Experience   32

Flipping Crucial Genetic Switches   34

The Ever-Alert Child   39

Contents

The Rattled Cage   40

The Difficulty of Not Knowing   43

The Sadness Seed   47

How Early Adversity Changes the Shape and Size of the Brain   49

The Inflamed Brain   50

A Perfect Storm: Childhood Stress, Brain Pruning, and
Adolescence   52

The Walking Wounded   57

The Really Good News   58

CHAPTER THREE: Why Do Some Suffer More than Others?   60

The Theory of Good Wobble   63

The Heavy Price We Pay for Secrets   67

The Power of Having Just One Reliable Adult   71

The Sensitivity Gene   75

The Perception Puzzle   81

Rashomon Revisited—or How We Remember   83

CHAPTER FOUR: The Female Brain on Adversity: The Link
to Autoimmune Disease, Depression, and Anxiety   89

Girls, Early Adversity, and the Autoimmune Connection   97

A Girl's Brain Is a Vulnerable Brain—in Unique Ways   104

Girls and the Genetic Link Between Childhood Adversity
and Adult Depression   110

CHAPTER FIVE: The Good Enough Family   114

When You Hope to Be a Better Parent than Your
Parents Were   115

The Reactive Parent   119

Contents

It's Hard to Give What Your Brain Never Received   122

How Children Absorb Their Parents' Stress   124

Parental Stress Translates into a Child's Pain   127

Nonparental Stressors: School and Friends   129

Early Biology Affects Later Relationships   134

The Neurobiology of Love   137

Attachment to Others Is a Biological Process   141

PART II

Recovering from Post Childhood Adversity Syndrome: How Do We Come Back to Who We Really Are?

CHAPTER SIX: Beginning Your Healing Journey   149

A Healing Journey: Twelve Steps to Help You Come Back to
Who You Really Are   151

    1. Take the ACE Survey   151

    2. Find Out Your Resilience Score   154

    3. Write to Heal   157

    4. Draw It   160

    5. Mindfulness Meditation—the Best Method for
      Repairing the Brain   161

    6. Tai Chi and Qigong   169

    7. Mindsight   170

    8. Loving-kindness   172

    9. Forgiveness   174

    10. Mending the Body, Moving the Body   177

    11. Managing the Mind Through the Gut   181

    12. Only Connect   184

Contents

CHAPTER SEVEN: Seeking Professional Help to Heal from
Post Childhood Adversity Syndrome   186

   1. Therapy Matters   186

   2. Somatic Experiencing   188

   3. Guided Imagery, Creative Visualization, and Hypnosis   192

   4. Neurofeedback   197

   5. EMDR and Desensitizing Memory   198

CHAPTER EIGHT: Parenting Well When You Haven't Been
Well Parented: Fourteen Strategies to Help You
Help Your Children   204

   1. Manage Your Own "Baggage"   207

   2. Don't Confuse Chronic Unpredictable Toxic Stress
      with Childhood Challenges that Foster Resilience   207

   3. Instill the Four S's in Your Children   210

   4. Look into Your Child's Eyes   210

   5. If You Lose It, Apologize—Right Away   211

   6. Validate and Normalize All of Your Child's Emotions   212

   7. Amplify the Good Feelings   213

   8. Stop, Look, Go   215

   9. Give a Name to Difficult Emotions   216

   10. The Incredible Power of the Twenty-Second Hug   217

   11. Make "What's Happening" a Safe and Open Conversation   217

   12. Reframe Stories of Intergenerational Trauma   219

   13. A Child Needs a Reliable Adult or Mentor   220

   14. Bring Mindfulness into Schools   223

IN CONCLUSION   227

   New Medical Horizons   228

   Hopeful Frontiers in Pediatric Medicine   232

Contents

LET'S CONTINUE THE CONVERSATION ABOUT ADVERSE
   CHILDHOOD EXPERIENCES   235

ACKNOWLEDGMENTS   237

NOTES   241

RESOURCES AND FURTHER READING   267

INDEX   269

INTRODUCTION

This book explores how the experiences of childhood shape us into the adults we become. Cutting-edge research tells us that what doesn't kill you doesn't necessarily make you stronger. Far more often, the opposite is true: the early chronic unpredictable stressors, losses, and adversities we face as children shape our biology in ways that predetermine our adult health. This early biological blueprint depicts our proclivity to develop life-altering adult illnesses such as heart disease, cancer, autoimmune disease, fibromyalgia, and depression. It also lays the groundwork for how we relate to others, how successful our love relationships will be, and how well we will nurture and raise our own children.

My own investigation into the relationship between childhood adversity and adult physical health began after I'd spent more than a dozen years struggling to manage several life-limiting autoimmune illnesses while raising young children and working as a journalist. In my forties, I was paralyzed twice with an autoimmune disease known as Guillain-Barré syndrome, similar to multiple sclerosis, but with a more sudden onset. I had muscle weakness; pervasive numbness; a pacemaker for vasovagal syncope, a fainting and seizing disorder; white and red blood cell counts so low my doctor suspected a problem was brewing in my bone marrow; and thyroid disease.

Still I knew: I was fortunate to be alive, and I was determined to live the fullest life possible. If the muscles in my hands didn't cooperate, I clasped an oversized pencil in my fist to write. If I couldn't get up the stairs because my legs resisted, I sat down halfway up and rested. I gutted through days battling flulike fatigue—pushing away fears about what might happen to my body next; faking it through work phone calls while lying prone on the floor; reserving what energy I had for moments with my children, husband, and family life; pretending that our "normal" was really okay by me. It had to be—there was no alternative in sight.

Increasingly, I devoted my skills as a science journalist to helping women with chronic illness, writing about the intersection between neuroscience, our immune systems, and the innermost workings of our human hearts. I investigated the many triggers of disease, reporting on chemicals in our environment and foods, genetics, and how inflammatory stress undermines our health. I reported on how going green, eating clean, and practices like mind-body meditation can help us to recuperate and recover. At health conferences I lectured to patients, doctors, and scientists. My mission became to do all I could to help readers who were caught in a chronic cycle of suffering, inflammation, or pain to live healthier, better lives.

In the midst of that quest, three years ago, in 2012, I came across a growing body of science based on a groundbreaking public health research study, the Adverse Childhood Experiences Study, or ACE Study. The ACE Study shows a clear scientific link between many types of childhood adversity and the adult onset of physical disease and mental health disorders. These traumas include being verbally put down and humiliated; being emotionally or physically neglected; being physically or sexually abused; living with a depressed parent, a parent with a mental illness, or a parent who is addicted to alcohol or other substances; witnessing one's mother being abused; and losing a parent to separation or divorce. The ACE Study measured ten types of adversity, but new research tells us that other types of childhood trauma—such as losing a parent to death, witnessing a sibling being abused, violence in one's community, growing up in poverty, witnessing a father being abused by a mother, being bullied by a classmate or teacher—also have a long-term impact.

These types of chronic adversities change the architecture of a child's brain, altering the expression of genes that control stress hormone output, triggering an overactive inflammatory stress response for life, and predisposing the child to adult disease. ACE research shows that 64 percent of adults faced one ACE in their childhood, and 40 percent faced two or more.

My own doctor at Johns Hopkins medical institutions confessed to me that she suspected that, given the chronic stress I'd faced in my childhood, my body and brain had been marinating in toxic inflammatory chemicals my whole life—predisposing me to the diseases I now faced.

My own story was a simple one of loss. When I was a girl, my father died suddenly. My family struggled and became estranged from our previously tight-knit, extended family. I had been exceptionally close to my father and I had looked to him for my sense of being safe, okay, and valued in the world. In every photo of our family, I'm smiling, clasped in his arms. When he died, childhood suddenly ended, overnight. If I am honest with myself, looking back, I cannot recall a single "happy memory" from there on out in my childhood. It was no one's fault. It just was. And I didn't dwell on any of that. In my mind, people who dwelled on their past, and especially on their childhood, were emotionally suspect.

I soldiered on. Life catapulted forward. I created a good life, worked hard as a science journalist to help meaningful causes, married a really good husband, and brought up children I adored—children I worked hard to stay alive for. But other than enjoying the lovely highlights of a hard-won family life, or being with close friends, I was pushing away pain. I felt myself a stranger at life's party. My body never let me forget that inside, pretend as I might, I had been masking a great deal of loss for a very long time. I felt myself to be "not like other people."

Seen through the lens of the new field of research into Adverse Childhood Experiences, it suddenly seemed almost predictable that, by the time I was in my early forties, my health would deteriorate and I would be brought—in my case, quite literally—to my knees.

Like many people, I was surprised, even dubious, when I first learned about ACEs and heard that so much of what we experience as adults is so inextricably linked to our childhood experiences. I did not consider myself to be someone who had had Adverse Childhood Experiences. But when I took the ACEs questionnaire and discovered my own ACE Score, my story also began to make so much more sense to me. This science was entirely new, but it also supported old ideas that we have long known to be true: "the child is father of the man." This research also told me that none of us is alone in our suffering.

One hundred thirty-three million Americans suffer from chronic illness and 116 million suffer from chronic pain. This revelation of the link between childhood adversity and adult illness can inform all of our efforts to heal. With this knowledge, physicians, health practitioners, psychologists, and psychiatrists can better understand their patients and find new insights to help them. And this knowledge will help us ensure that the children in our lives—whether we are parents, mentors, teachers, or coaches—don't suffer from the long-term consequences of these sorts of adversity.

To learn everything I could, I spent two years interviewing the leading scientists who research and study the effects of Adverse Childhood Experiences and toxic childhood stress. I combed through seventy research papers that comprise the ACE Study and hundreds of other studies from our nation's best research institutions that support and complement these findings. And I followed thirteen individuals who suffered early adversity and later faced adult health struggles, who were able to forge their own life-changing paths to physical and emotional healing.

In these pages, I explore the damage that Adverse Childhood Experiences can do to the brain and body; how these invisible changes contribute to the development of disease including autoimmune diseases, long into adulthood; why some individuals are more likely to be affected by early adversity than others; why girls and women are more affected than men; and how early adversity affects our ability to love and parent.

Just as important, I explore how we can reverse the effects of early toxic stress on our biology, and come back to being who we really are. I hope to help readers to avoid spending so much of their lives locked in pain.

Some points to bear in mind as you read these pages:

- Adverse Childhood Experiences should not be confused with the inevitable small challenges of childhood that create resilience. There are many normal moments in a happy childhood, when things don't go a child's way, when parents lose it and apologize, when children fail and learn to try again. Adverse Childhood Experiences are very different sorts of experiences; they are scary, chronic, unpredictable stressors, and often a child does not have the adult support needed to help navigate safely through them.

- Adverse Childhood Experiences are linked to a far greater likelihood of illness in adulthood, but they are not the only factor. All disease is multifactorial. Genetics, exposures to toxins, and infection all play a role. But for those who have experienced ACEs and toxic stress, other disease-promoting factors become more damaging. To use a simple metaphor, imagine the immune system as being something like a barrel. If you encounter too many environmental toxins from chemicals, a poor processed-food diet, viruses, infections, and chronic or acute stressors in adulthood, your barrel will slowly fill. At some point, there may be one certain exposure, that last drop that causes the barrel to spill over and disease to develop. Having faced the chronic unpredictable stressors of Adverse Childhood Experiences is a lot like starting life with your barrel half full. ACEs are not the only factor in determining who will develop disease later in life. But they may make it more likely that one will.

- The research into Adverse Childhood Experiences has some factors in common with the research on post-traumatic stress disorder, or PTSD. But childhood adversity can lead to a far wider range of physical and emotional health consequences than the overt symptoms of post-traumatic stress. They are not the same.

- The Adverse Childhood Experiences of extreme poverty and neighborhood violence are not addressed specifically in the original research. Yet clearly, growing up in unsafe neighborhoods where there is poverty and gang violence or in a war-torn area anywhere around the world creates toxic childhood stress, and that relationship is now being more deeply studied. It is an important field of inquiry and one I do not attempt to address here; that is a different book, but one that is no less important.

- Adverse Childhood Experiences are not an excuse for egregious behavior. They should not be considered a "blame the childhood" moral pass. The research allows us to finally tackle real and lasting physical and emotional change from an entirely new vantage point, but it is not about making excuses.

- This research is not an invitation to blame parents. Adverse Childhood Experiences are often an intergenerational legacy, and patterns of neglect, maltreatment, and adversity almost always originate many generations prior to one's own.

The new science on Adverse Childhood Experiences and toxic stress has given us a new lens through which to understand the human story; why we suffer; how we parent, raise, and mentor our children; how we might better prevent, treat, and manage illness in our medical care system; and how we can recover and heal on a deeper level than we thought possible.

And that last bit is the best news of all. The brain, which is so changeable in childhood, remains malleable throughout life. Today researchers around the world have discovered a range of powerful ways to reverse the damage that Adverse Childhood Experiences do to both brain and body. No matter how old you are, or how old your children may be, there are scientifically supported and relatively simple steps that you can take to reboot the brain, create new pathways that promote healing, and come back to who it is you were meant to be.

To find out about how many categories of ACEs you might have faced when you were a child or teenager, and your own ACE Score, turn the page and take the Adverse Childhood Experiences Survey for yourself.

TAKE THE ADVERSE CHILDHOOD
EXPERIENCES (ACE) SURVEY

You may have picked up this book because you had a painful or traumatic childhood. You may suspect that your past has something to do with your current health problems, your depression, or your anxiety. Or perhaps you are reading this book because you are worried about the health of a spouse, partner, friend, parent—or even your own child—who has survived a trauma or suffered adverse experiences. In order to assess the likelihood that an Adverse Childhood Experience is affecting your health or the health of your loved one, please take a moment to fill out the following survey before you read this book.

ADVERSE CHILDHOOD EXPERIENCES SURVEY

Prior to your eighteenth birthday:

1. Did a parent or another adult in the household *often or very often* ... swear at you, insult you, put you down, or humiliate you? *Or* act in a way that made you afraid that you might be physically hurt?

   Yes   No

   If yes, enter 1 _____

2. Did a parent or another adult in the household *often or very often* ... push, grab, slap, or throw something at you? *Or* ever hit you so hard that you had marks or were injured?

   Yes No

   If yes, enter 1 _____

3. Did an adult or person at least five years older than you *ever* ... touch or fondle you or have you touch their body in a sexual way? *Or* attempt to touch you or touch you inappropriately or sexually abuse you?

   Yes No

   If yes, enter 1 _____

4. Did you *often or very often* feel that ... no one in your family loved you or thought you were important or special? *Or* feel that your family members didn't look out for one another, feel close to one another, or support one another?

   Yes No

   If yes, enter 1 _____

5. Did you *often or very often* feel that ... you didn't have enough to eat, had to wear dirty clothes, and had no one to protect you? *Or* that your parents were too drunk or high to take care of you or take you to the doctor if you needed it?

   Yes No

   If yes, enter 1 _____

6. Was a biological parent *ever* lost to you through divorce, abandonment, or another reason?

Yes   No

If yes, enter 1 _____

7. Was your mother or stepmother *often or very often* pushed, grabbed, slapped, or have something thrown at her? *Or was she sometimes, often, or very often* kicked, bitten, hit with a fist, or hit with something hard? *Or ever* repeatedly hit over the course of at least a few minutes or threatened with a gun or knife?

Yes   No

If yes, enter 1 _____

8. Did you live with anyone who was a problem drinker or alcoholic, or who used street drugs?

Yes   No

If yes, enter 1 _____

9. Was a household member depressed or mentally ill, or did a household member attempt suicide?

Yes   No

If yes, enter 1 _____

10. Did a household member go to prison?

Yes   No

If yes, enter 1 _____

Add up your "Yes" answers: _____ (this is your ACE Score)

Now take a moment and ask yourself how your experiences might be affecting your physical, emotional, and mental well-being. Is it possible that someone you love has been affected by Adverse Childhood Experiences they experienced? Are any children or young people you care for in adverse situations now?

Keep your Adverse Childhood Experiences Score in mind as you read the stories and science that follow, and keep your own experiences in mind, as well as those of the people you love. You may find this science to be the missing link in understanding why you or your loved one is having health problems. And this missing link will also lead to the information you will need in order to heal.

PART I

How It Is We Become Who We Are

CHAPTER ONE

Every Adult Was Once a Child

If you saw Laura walking down the New York City street where she lives today, you'd see a well-dressed forty-six-year-old woman with auburn hair and green eyes who exudes a sense of "I matter here." She looks entirely in charge of her life—as long as you don't see the small ghosts trailing after her.

When Laura was growing up, her mom was bipolar. Laura's mom had her good moments: she helped Laura with school projects, braided her hair, and taught her the name of every bird at the bird feeder. But when Laura's mom suffered from depressive bouts, she'd lock herself in her room for hours. At other times she was manic and hypercritical, which took its toll on everyone around her. Laura's dad, a vascular surgeon, was kind to Laura, but rarely around. He was, she says, "home late, out the door early—and then just plain out the door."

Laura recalls a family trip to the Grand Canyon when she was ten. In a photo taken that day, Laura and her parents sit on a bench, sporting tourist whites. The sky is blue and cloudless, and behind them the dark, ribboned shadows of the canyon stretch deep and wide. It is a perfect summer day.

"That afternoon my mom was teaching me to identify the ponderosa pines," Laura recalls. "Anyone looking at us would have assumed we were a normal, loving family." Then, something seemed to shift, as it sometimes would. Laura's parents began arguing about where to set up the tripod for their family photo. By the time the three of them sat down, her parents weren't speaking. As they put on fake smiles for the camera, Laura's mom suddenly pinched her daughter's midriff around the back rim of her shorts, and told her to stop "staring off into space." Then, a second pinch: "no wonder you're turning into a butterball, you ate so much cheesecake last night you're hanging over your shorts!"

If you look hard at Laura's face in the photograph, you can see that she's not squinting at the Arizona sun, but holding back tears.

When Laura was fifteen, her dad moved three states away with a new wife-to-be. He sent cards and money, but called less and less often. Her mother's untreated bipolar disorder worsened. Laura's days were punctuated with put-downs that caught her off guard as she walked across the living room. "My mom would spit out something like, 'You look like a semiwide from behind. If you're ever wondering why no boy asks you out, that's why!'" One of Laura's mother's recurring lines was, "You were such a pretty baby, I don't know what happened." Sometimes Laura recalls, "My mom would go on a vitriolic diatribe about my dad until spittle foamed on her chin. I'd stand there, trying not to hear her as she went on and on, my whole body shaking inside." Laura never invited friends over, for fear they'd find out her secret: her mom "wasn't like other moms."

Some thirty years later, Laura says, "In many ways, no matter where I go or what I do, I'm still in my mother's house." Today, "If a car swerves into my lane, a grocery store clerk is rude, my husband and I argue, or my boss calls me in to talk over a problem, I feel something flip over inside. It's like there's a match standing inside too near a flame, and with the smallest breeze, it ignites." Something, she says, "just doesn't feel right. Things feel bigger than they should be. Some days, I feel as if I'm living my life in an emotional boom box where the volume is turned up too high."

To see Laura, you would never know that she is "always shaking a little, only invisibly, deep down in my cells."

Laura's sense that something is wrong inside is mirrored by her physical health. In her midthirties, she began suffering from migraines that landed her in bed for days at a time. At forty, Laura developed an autoimmune thyroid disease. At forty-four, during a routine exam, Laura's doctor didn't like the sound of her heart. An EKG revealed an arrhythmia. An echocardiogram showed that Laura had a condition known as dilated cardiomyopathy. The left ventricle of her heart was weak; the muscle had trouble pumping blood into her heart. Next thing Laura knew, she was a heart disease patient, undergoing surgery. Today, Laura has a cardioverter defibrillator implanted in the left side of her chest to prevent heart failure. The two-inch scar from the implant is deceivingly small.

John's parents met in Asia when his father was deployed there as an army officer. After a whirlwind romance, his parents married and moved to the United States. For as long as John can remember, he says, "my parents' marriage was deeply troubled, as was my relationship with my dad. I consider myself to have been raised by my mom and her mom. I longed to feel a deeper connection with my dad, but it just wasn't there. He couldn't extend himself in that way."

John occasionally runs his hands through his short blond hair, as he carefully chooses his words. "My dad would get so worked up and pissed off about trivial things. He'd throw out opinions that we all knew were factually incorrect, and just keep arguing." If John's dad said the capital of New York was New York City, it didn't matter if John showed him it was Albany. "He'd ask me to help in the garage and I'd be doing everything right, and then a half hour into it I'd put the screwdriver down in the wrong spot and he'd start yelling and not let up. There was never any praise. Even when he was the one who'd made a mistake, it somehow became my fault. He could not be wrong about anything."

As John got older, it seemed wrong to him that "my dad was constantly pointing out all the mistakes that my brother and I made, without acknowledging any of his own." His dad chronically criticized his mother, who was, John says, "kinder and more confident."

When John was twelve, he interjected himself into the fights between his parents. One Christmas Eve, when he was fifteen, John awoke to the sound of "a scream and a commotion. I realized it was my mother screaming. I jumped out of bed and ran into my parents' room, shouting, 'What the hell is going on here?' My mother sputtered, 'He's choking me!' My father had his hands around my mother's neck. I yelled at him: 'You stay right here! Don't you dare move! Mom is coming with me!' I took my mother downstairs. She was sobbing. I was trying to understand what was happening, trying to be the adult between them."

Later that Christmas morning, John's father came down the steps to the living room where John and his mom were sleeping. "No one explained," he says. "My little brother came downstairs and we had Christmas morning as if nothing had happened."

Not long after, John's grandmother, "who'd been an enormous source of love for my mom and me," died suddenly. John says, "It was a terrible shock and loss for both of us. My father couldn't support my mom or me in our grieving. He told my mom, 'You just need to get over it!' He was the quintessential narcissist. If it wasn't about him, it wasn't important, it wasn't happening."

Today, John is a boyish forty. He has warm hazel eyes and a wide, affable grin that would be hard not to warm up to. But beneath his easy, open demeanor, John struggles with an array of chronic illnesses.

By the time John was thirty-three, his blood pressure was shockingly high for a young man. He began to experience bouts of stabbing stomach pain and diarrhea and often had blood in his stool. These episodes grew more frequent. He had a headache every day of his life. By thirty-four, he'd developed chronic fatigue, and was so wiped out that sometimes he struggled to make it through an entire day at work.

For years, John had loved to go hiking to relieve stress, but by the time he was thirty-five, he couldn't muster the physical stamina. "One day it hit me, 'I'm still a young man and I'll never go hiking again.'"

John's relationships, like his physical body, were never quite healthy. John remembers falling deeply in love in his early thirties. After dating his girlfriend for a year, she invited him to meet her family. During his stay with them, John says, "I became acutely aware of how different I was from kids who grew up without the kind of shame and blame I endured." One night, his girlfriend, her sisters, and their boyfriends all decided to go out dancing. "Everyone was sitting around the dinner table planning this great night out and I remember looking around at her family and the only thing going through my mind were these words: 'I do *not* belong here.' Everyone seemed so normal and happy. I was horrified suddenly at the idea of trying to play along and pretend that I knew how to be part of a happy family."

So John faked "being really tired. My girlfriend was sweet and stayed with me and we didn't go. She kept asking what was wrong and at some point I just started crying and I couldn't stop. She wanted to help, but instead of telling her how insecure I was, or asking for her reassurance, I told her I was crying because I wasn't in love with her."

John's girlfriend was, he says, "completely devastated." She drove John to a hotel that night. "She and her family were shocked. No one could understand what had happened." Even though John had been deeply in love, his fear won out. "I couldn't let her find out how crippled I was by the shame and grief I carried inside."

Bleeding from his inflamed intestines, exhausted by chronic fatigue, debilitated and distracted by pounding headaches, often struggling with work, and unable to feel comfortable in a relationship, John was stuck in a universe of pain and solitude, and he couldn't get out.

—

Georgia's childhood seems far better than the norm: she had two living parents who stayed married through thick and thin, and they lived in a stunning home with walls displaying Ivy League diplomas; Georgia's father was a well-respected, Yale-educated investment banker. Her mom stayed at home with Georgia and two younger sisters. The five of them appear, in photos, to be the perfect family.

All *seemed* fine, growing up, practically perfect.

"But I felt, very early on, that something wasn't quite right in our home, and that no one was talking about it," Georgia says. "Our house was saturated by a kind of unease all the time. You could never put your finger on what it was, but it was there."

Georgia's mom was "emotionally distant and controlling," Georgia recalls. "If you said or did something she didn't like, she had a way of going stone cold right in front of you—she'd become what I used to think of as a moving statue that looked like my mother, only she wouldn't look at you or speak to you." The hardest part was that Georgia never knew what she'd done wrong. "I just knew that I was shut out of her world until whenever she decided I was worth speaking to again."

For instance, her mother would "give my sisters and me a tiny little tablespoon of ice cream and then say, 'You three will just have to share that.' We knew better than to complain. If we did, she'd tell us how ungrateful we were, and suddenly she wouldn't speak to us."

Georgia's father was a borderline alcoholic and "would occasionally just blow up over nothing," she says. "One time he was changing a lightbulb and he just started cursing and screaming because it broke. He had these unpredictable eruptions of rage. They were rare but unforgettable." Georgia was so frightened at times that "I'd run like a dog with my tail between my legs to hide until it was safe to come out again."

Georgia was "so sensitive to the shifting vibe in our house that I could tell when my father was about to erupt before even he knew. The air would get so tight and I'd know—it's going to happen again." The worst part was that "We had to pretend my father's outbursts weren't happening. He'd scream about something minor, and then he'd go take a nap. Or you'd hear him strumming his guitar in his den."

Between her mother's silent treatments and her dad's tirades, Georgia spent much of her childhood trying to anticipate and move out of the way of her parents' anger. She had the sense, even when she was nine or ten, "that their anger was directed at each other. They didn't fight, but there was a constant low hum of animosity between them. At times it seemed they vehemently hated each other." Once, fearing that her inebriated father would crash his car after an argument with her mother, Georgia stole his car keys and refused to give them back.

Today, at age forty-nine, Georgia is reflective about her childhood. "I internalized all the emotions that were storming around me in my house, and in some ways it's as if I've carried all that external angst inside me all my life." Over the decades, carrying that pain has exacted a high toll. At first, Georgia says, "My physical pain began as a low whisper in my body." But by the time she entered Columbia graduate school to pursue a PhD in classics, "I'd started having severe back problems. I was in so much physical pain, I could not sit in a chair. I had to study lying down." At twenty-six, Georgia was diagnosed with degenerative disc disease. "My body just started screaming with its pain."

Over the next few years, in addition to degenerative disc disease, Georgia was diagnosed with severe depression, adrenal fatigue—and finally, fibromyalgia. "I've spent my adult life in doctors' clinics and trying various medications to relieve my pain," she says. "But there is no relief in sight."

———

Laura's, John's, and Georgia's life stories illustrate the physical price we pay, as adults, for childhood adversity. New findings in neuroscience, psychology, and medicine have recently unveiled the exact ways in which childhood adversity biologically alters us for life. This groundbreaking research tells us that the emotional trauma we face when we are young has farther-reaching consequences than we might have imagined. Adverse Childhood Experiences change the architecture of our brains and the health of our immune systems, they trigger and sustain inflammation in both body and brain, and they influence our overall physical health and longevity long into adulthood. These physical changes, in turn, prewrite the story of how we will react to the world around us, and how well we will work, and parent, befriend, and love other people throughout the course of our adult lives.

This is true whether our childhood wounds are deeply traumatic, such as witnessing violence in our family, as John did; or more chronic living-room variety humiliations, such as those Laura endured; or more private but pervasive familial dysfunctions, such as Georgia's.

All of these Adverse Childhood Experiences can lead to deep biophysical changes in a child that profoundly alter the developing brain and immunology in ways that also change the health of the adult he or she will become.

Scientists have come to this startling understanding of the link between Adverse Childhood Experiences and later physical illness in adulthood thanks, in large part, to the work of two individuals: a dedicated physician in San Diego, and a determined medical epidemiologist from the Centers for Disease Control (CDC). Together, during the 1980s and 1990s—the same years when Laura, John, and Georgia were growing up—these two researchers slowly uncovered the stunning scientific link between Adverse Childhood Experiences and later physical and neurological inflammation and life-changing adult health outcomes.

The Philosophical Physicians

In 1985 physician and researcher Vincent J. Felitti, MD, chief of a revolutionary preventive care initiative at the Kaiser Permanente Medical

Program in San Diego, noticed a startling pattern: adult patients who were obese also alluded to traumatic incidents in their childhood.

Felitti came to this realization almost by accident. In the mid-1980s, a significant number of patients in Kaiser Permanente's obesity program were, with the help and support of Felitti and his nurses, successfully losing hundreds of pounds a year nonsurgically, a remarkable feat. The program seemed a resounding success, up until a large number of patients who were losing substantial amounts of weight began to drop out. The attrition rate didn't make sense, and Felitti was determined to find out what was going on. He conducted face-to-face interviews with 286 patients. In the course of Felitti's one-on-one conversations, a striking number of patients confided that they had faced trauma in their childhood; many had been sexually abused. To these patients, eating was a solution: it soothed the anxiety, fear, and depression that they had secreted away inside for decades. Their weight served, too, as a shield against unwanted physical attention, and they didn't want to let it go.

Felitti's conversations with this large group of patients allowed him to perceive a pattern—and a new way of looking at human health and well-being—that other physicians just were not seeing. It became clear to him that, for his patients, obesity, "though an obvious physical sign," was not the core problem to be treated, "any more than smoke is the core problem to be treated in house fires."

In 1990, Felitti presented his findings at a national obesity conference. He told the group of physicians gathered that he believed "certain of our intractable public health problems" had root causes hidden "by shame, by secrecy, and by social taboos against exploring certain areas of life experience."

Although Felitti's peers blasted him for his presentation—one stood up in the audience and accused Felitti of offering "excuses" for patients' "failed lives"—Felitti was unfazed. At that conference, a colleague and epidemiologist from the CDC advised Felitti that if what he was saying was true, it had enormous import for medicine in general.

He suggested that Felitti set up a study with thousands of patients suffering from all types of diseases, not just obesity. Felitti agreed. Indeed, he suspected that a wide-scale study would reveal a larger societal health pattern: a link between many types of childhood adversity and the likelihood of developing a range of serious adult health problems.

Felitti joined forces with the CDC. At that time, the Health Appraisal Division of Kaiser Permanente's Department of Preventive Medicine was providing unusually comprehensive medical exams and evaluations to fifty-eight thousand adults a year. One of the CDC's medical epidemiologists, Robert Anda, MD, who had been researching the relationship between coronary heart disease and depression, visited the clinic in San Diego. And he recommended that Felitti turn it into a national epidemiology laboratory. With such a vast patient cohort, they might be able to discover if patients who experienced different types of adverse experiences in childhood were more likely to suffer from adult diseases such as heart disease, autoimmune disease, and cancer.

Felitti and Anda asked twenty-six thousand patients who came through the department "if they would be interested in helping us understand how childhood events might affect adult health," says Felitti. More than seventeen thousand agreed.

Drawing upon Felitti's original 286 interviews, Anda conceptualized and designed a new study, adding additional survey questions to Felitti's existing patient questionnaires. These questions focused on ten types of adversity, or Adverse Childhood Experiences (ACEs), and probed into patients' childhood and adolescent histories.

The first five questions were personal; they had to do with emotional and physical stressors a patient might have faced as a child or teenager. These included having had a parent who insulted, humiliated, or made the child feel emotionally afraid; hit, pushed, or slapped them; or touched them sexually. These questions also included feeling that no one in the family thought the patient was important or that the family members didn't look out for one another; feeling there was no one to provide protection; or being neglected to the point of not having clean clothes or enough food, or not being taken to the doctor when ill.

The next five questions had to do with other family members—the specifics of one's household situation while growing up: loss of a parent due to separation or divorce; witnessing one's mother being hit, grabbed, threatened or beaten; someone in the home suffering from alcoholism or another addiction; someone in the home suffering from depression or another mental or behavioral health problem, or being suicidal; or a family member being sent to prison. After the interviews, each participant in Felitti and Anda's study was assigned an ACE Score corresponding to the number of categories of adverse or traumatic events he or she had experienced while young.

In one way or another, all ten questions spoke to family dysfunction.

And with these ten questions, the Adverse Childhood Experiences Study was born.

———

If you have also taken the Adverse Childhood Experiences questionnaire for yourself, now might be an excellent time to turn back to it on page xxi. It might prove helpful to you in further understanding yourself and your health.

Time Does Not Heal All Wounds

The patients Felitti and Anda surveyed were not troubled or disadvantaged; the average patient was fifty-seven, and three-quarters were college educated. These were "successful" men and women with good educations, mostly white, middle class, with health benefits and stable jobs. The scientist expected that the number of "yes" answers on the Adverse Childhood Experiences Survey would be fairly low.

But the number of "yes" answers turned out to be far higher than anyone had predicted. Two-thirds—64 percent—of participants answered yes to one or more categories, meaning they had experienced at least one of these forms of childhood adversity before turning eighteen. And 87 percent of those who answered yes to one ACE question also had additional Adverse Childhood Experiences. Forty percent had experienced two or more categories of Adverse Childhood Experiences, and 12.5 percent had an ACE Score of 4 or more.

Only a third of participants had an ACE Score of zero.

Felitti and Anda wanted to find out whether there was a correlation between the number of categories of Adverse Childhood Experiences each individual had faced and the degree of illness and physical disorders he or she developed as an adult.

Indeed, the correlation proved so powerful that Anda was not only "stunned," but deeply moved.

"I wept," Anda says. "I saw how much people had suffered and I wept."

Felitti was also deeply affected. "Our findings exceeded anything we had conceived. The correlation between having a difficult childhood and facing illness as an adult offered a whole new lens through which we could view human heath and disease."

Here, says Felitti, "was the missing piece as to what was causing so much of our unspoken suffering as human beings."

How many categories of Adverse Childhood Experiences patients had encountered could by and large predict how much medical care they would require in adulthood: the higher one's ACE Score, the higher the number of doctor visits they'd had in the past year, and the higher their number of unexplained physical symptoms.

People with an ACE Score of 4 were twice as likely to be diagnosed with cancer than someone with an ACE Score of 0. For each ACE Score an individual had, the chance of being hospitalized with an autoimmune disease in adulthood rose 20 percent. Someone with an ACE

Score of 4 was 460 percent more likely to be facing depression than someone with a score of 0.

An ACE Score of 6 and higher shortened an individual's life-span by almost twenty years.

Felitti and Anda wondered if they were finding this strong correlation because individuals who had been traumatized in childhood were more likely to smoke, drink, and overeat as a sort of self-coping strategy to manage chronic anxiety—and this accounted for their poorer health. But while these unhealthy coping mechanisms were common, they were not the main explanation. For instance, those with ACE Scores of 7 or higher who didn't drink or smoke, and who weren't overweight, diabetic, and didn't have high cholesterol, still had a 360 percent higher risk of heart disease than those with an ACE Score of 0.

The chronic stress of emotional or physical adversity these adults had experienced when they were growing up was making them ill decades later—even though they had healthy habits and lifestyles. In a few years (as we will see in Chapter Two) scientists would discover the precise mechanisms by which this early stress converted into biomedical disease. But the overall pattern was undeniable.

"Time," says Felitti, "does not heal all wounds. One does not 'just get over' something—not even fifty years later." Instead, he says, "Time conceals. And human beings convert traumatic emotional experiences in childhood into organic disease later in life."

Often, these illnesses can be chronic and lifelong. Autoimmune disease. Heart disease. Chronic bowel disorders. Migraines. Persistent depression. Even today, doctors puzzle over these very conditions: why are they so prevalent; why are some patients more prone to them than others; and why are they so difficult to treat?

——

At seventy-nine, Felliti has a full head of silver hair and salt-and-pepper eyebrows, and has, with Adna, coauthored seventy-four more papers based on the Adverse Childhood Experiences Study. He and

Anda are widely regarded as the scientific fathers of the extensive body of research that has led to a global understanding that adverse childhood events can change people's biology and lead to chronic illness and negative health effects over their life-span. Today, more than 1,500 studies cite ACE research and the World Health Organization now utilizes the Adverse Childhood Experiences questionnaire in fourteen countries to help screen for emotional distress and trauma that might lead to poor health. In the United States, twenty-nine states and Washington, DC, are using the ACE questionnaire to help improve public health.

The more research that's done, the more granular details emerge about the profound link between adverse experiences and adult disease. Scientists at Duke, the University of California, San Francisco, and Brown have shown that childhood adversity damages us on a cellular level in ways that prematurely age our cells and affect our longevity. Adults who faced early life stress show greater erosion in what's known as telomeres—which are protective caps that sit on the ends of strands of DNA to keep DNA healthy and intact. As telomeres erode, we're more likely to develop disease, and we age faster. As our telomeres age and expire, our cells expire, and eventually, so do we.

Researchers have also seen a correlation between specific types of Adverse Childhood Experiences and a range of diseases. For instance, children whose parents die, or who face emotional or physical abuse, or experience childhood neglect, or witness marital discord between their parents are more likely to develop cardiovascular disease, lung disease, diabetes, headaches, multiple sclerosis, and lupus as adults. They are more likely to develop cancer or have a stroke. Facing difficult circumstances in childhood increases sixfold your chances of having chronic fatigue syndrome, also known as myalgic encephalomyelitis, as an adult. Kids who lose a parent have triple the risk of depression as adults. Children whose parents divorce are twice as likely to suffer a stroke at some point in their lifetime.

The Body Remembers—and Will Tell Its Tale

Kat was five years old when her mom left her father. Her mom had good reason to end her marriage. Kat recalls that during one of her parents' arguments, "my father ripped my mom's glasses off her face, threw them on the ground, and crushed them under his heel."

One day, Kat's mom drove her to her father's carpet-cleaning business. When they arrived, her mother told her to stay put in the "way way back" of their wood-paneled station wagon. "I'll be back in a minute," she told her five-year-old daughter. "I need to talk to your father." Kat remembers lying there happily and coloring in a book. Sometime later, Kat thought she heard a scream. Startled, she looked up and realized that her mom wasn't back. She didn't know how much time had passed, but she was hot, hungry, and suddenly wanted her mom. She climbed out of the car and walked to the building. The front door was locked, so Kat walked over to the side window and stood on her tippytoes to see inside for any sign of her mom or dad.

Beyond the lobby, she could see the glass door to her father's office. Through it, she saw her mother's feet and ankles on the floor—"as if she were facedown on the carpet. She wasn't moving. So I tried the door but it was locked. I tried it again. No one heard me. No one came. I ran back to the station wagon and locked myself inside."

When her father came out to the car a few minutes later, he told her, "Your mom got caught up on the phone, Kitty." He smiled and said, "I'm taking you to my place." Kat got out of the station wagon and into her dad's car. "As he drove us to his town house, he kept smiling at me as if everything was great."

Kat still has the news clippings and TV footage from back then: the police suspected her father of killing her mother, but they didn't have a body. When her mother's station wagon was found across town, the upholstery was spotless, as was the carpet in her dad's office.

Detectives asked Kat to replay the scene with Barbie and Ken dolls and had her testify in court to say exactly what she'd witnessed. She climbed onto the stand, "clutching my Care Bear, answering everyone's questions," Kat says. "My dad was looking at me from across the courtroom with puppy dog eyes, as if to say, 'Kitty, you know I could never have hurt anyone.'" But, Kat says, "I'd think back to that moment when I'd seen my mom's feet lying there, how she wasn't moving, how she never came back for me, and I knew that something terrible had happened."

Kat provided testimony that convinced the jury, who sent her dad away to jail.

Kat was eight years old when her dad wrote a letter from prison, confessing his crime to the *Washington Post* and spelling out many of the gory details: he'd removed Kat's mom's head, crushed her skull and teeth, and thrown them into the Potomac River. He'd buried her body and used his carpet cleaning machines to scrub the car and office until they were spotless.

When detectives found the grave, they discovered what bones remained of Kat's mother's body, but because her father had been sentenced for manslaughter, he could not be tried for the same crime again after he'd confessed. He would serve only ten years for manslaughter instead of remaining in prison for life for first-degree murder.

Kat's family held a second funeral. "First we had a funeral with no body," Kat says. "Then we had a viewing of my mother's bones. My family had me look at my mom's remains so that I would know that she hadn't just 'disappeared.' She was really gone. I just stood there, staring at my mother's lonely, white bones—without her skull. There was nothing left of the mom I had loved, the mom who'd loved me."

Kat and I are sitting at the dark wooden upstairs bar at the Metropolitan in Baltimore's historic Federal Hill. After she describes seeing her mother's bones, we are both quiet for several minutes.

It is an early October evening, and the air outside is soft, gently

18

holding on to an Indian summer, a full moon in the indigo sky. Inside, the bar's dark paneling and crumbly brick walls seem a fitting backdrop for a ghost story. And in a sense Kat's story is just that: the story of a woman whose past haunted her entire life, a woman who, now thirty-seven, longs to be free of her ghosts, the living and the dead.

For the rest of Kat's childhood, she moved from one relative's house to another's, up and down the East Coast, living in four homes before entering high school. Finally, in high school, she lived for a few years with her grandmother, her mom's mom, whom she called "G-Ma." No one ever talked about her mom's murder. "In my family, my past was 'The Big Unmentionable'—including my role in putting my own father in jail," she says. In high school, Kat appeared to be doing well. She was an honor student who played four varsity sports. Beneath the surface, however, "I was secretly self-medicating with alcohol because otherwise, by the time everything stopped and it got quiet at night, I could not sleep, I would just lie there and a terrible panic would overtake me."

She went to college, failed out, went back, and graduated. She went to work in advertising, and one day, dissatisfied, quit. She went back to grad school, piling up debt. She became a teacher. Kat quit that job too, when a relationship she had formed with another teacher imploded. At the age of thirty-four, Kat went to stay with her brother and his family in Hawaii. She got a job as a valet, parking cars. "I'd come home from parking cars all day and curl up on my bed in the back bedroom of my brother's house, and lie there feeling desperate and alone, my heart beating with anxiety."

She decided to go back to the East Coast, and settled in Brooklyn, New York, where she took a job as a bartender.

"If there was a ground zero, that was it," Kat says. "I was thirty-four-years old, with a master's degree, valeting cars, bartending. I was a walking specter of human sadness. I couldn't calm myself down. All I could see was that no matter how hard I tried to change my life, life was going nowhere for me. I never felt okay in the world."

Then the toxic emotional stress of Kat's childhood began to show up in physical ways. It was as if that decades-old pain began to bubble up to the surface. Rashes appeared all over Kat's skin—across her hands, legs, and stomach. Photos taken at that time show red, open, oozing sores covering almost her entire body.

"I was in so much physical pain," Kat says. "I couldn't sleep. I couldn't turn over. I couldn't stop scratching." At the end of each day, she says, "My clothes would be stuck to all my wet, raw sores. I'd have to peel my pants off my body. It was agonizing."

The first doctor Kat saw put her on a heavy dose of prednisone. But her symptoms worsened. "My joints became enlarged and swollen," she says.

Every day Kat would bike to her bartending job. "But I had to pedal my bike with one foot," Kat says. "One knee was so swollen and inflamed, I couldn't bend it at all."

Kat saw another doctor and then another to find out what was causing so much fiery inflammation in her skin and joints. Blood tests showed that her white blood cell count was so low that she was fighting an issue in her bone marrow. Kat's autoantibody count was unusually high. It looked as if she had connective tissue disease, possibly lupus, or rheumatoid arthritis.

Kat saw a few more doctors, searching for holistic solutions in addition to traditional care. And then one doctor, after asking about her family and life history, asked a question that would change Kat's life forever. She asked her, "Have you thought about the relationship between the high level of emotional stress you went through thirty years ago and your level of physical inflammation now?"

"That completely surprised me," Kat says. She understood why she might have a hard time feeling happy as an adult, given what she'd been through growing up. But she never imagined that there could be a physiological connection "between what happened when I was five, and my immune system breaking down thirty years later."

Then her doctor pointed out one detail that Kat had completely overlooked. It floored her. "You said your mom was murdered when she was thirty-five," her doctor said, peering at Kat's chart, noting her birth date. "It's almost your birthday. In a few weeks you'll be turning thirty-five. You're coming up to the exact age your mom was when she was murdered by your father."

That was a huge "aha moment for me," Kat says. "I'd never considered the possibility of a link between what I'd faced as a kid and my own physical breakdown. But something inside me knew, deep inside, that what she was saying was true."

"It was as if I'd been running from my past, my story, my pain, and I'd run smack into myself again," she says.

All that emotional suffering and toxic stress had been wreaking havoc in Kat's mind and heart—and in her body, too.

Kat combs her fingers, separated like a V, through her dark, boyish bangs, pushing them back to reveal light brown eyes. "I felt a sense of relief that I had this clue into what was going on with me. But the more I thought about what my doctor said, I also felt grief. I had to ask myself, 'Who might I be now if I hadn't faced so much pain and sadness back then?'"

Would she have had a very different life if she'd had a happier childhood?

Could she find her way back to the healthier person she might have been if she hadn't suffered such trauma early on?

Kat began to focus on one overarching question: "How can I make sure that my broken, scarred self doesn't win out over who I want to become in my life?"

———

Like the stories of adversity for Laura, John, and Georgia, Kat's story illustrates that the past can tick away inside us for decades like a silent time bomb, until it sets off a cellular message that lets us know the body does not forget the past.

—

Kat would be given one point in her Adverse Childhood Experiences Score for each of the following categories of family dysfunction that she experienced: (1) she often felt that no one in her family loved her or thought she was important or special, and that none of her family members looked out for one another; (2) she often felt there was no one to protect her or look out for her; (3) Kat witnessed her mother being threatened (and was an unknowing witness to her murder); and (4) Kat had an immediate family member—her dad—who went to prison.

And finally, (5) Kat would be given an additional point in her ACE Score for having lost her parents.

In other words, Kat has a very high ACE Score of 5.

And yet if you had met Kat at twenty or thirty, it's unlikely that you would have recognized the link between her childhood trauma and the many adult health—and life—hurdles that would later challenge her.

Her bosses would simply have thought that she sabotaged her own talent, limiting her career possibilities. Her friends during those years might have described her as manipulative, overreactive, and, as Kat says, "quick to cast myself as the victim and blame other people in even small misunderstandings." Most physicians didn't ask Kat anything about her childhood, beyond her family history of cancer and heart disease. They were more likely to suggest the newest, most promising antidepressants, anxiety meds, steroids, or immune suppressants— hoping that pills and creams alone would improve her symptoms.

But the trauma that Kat experienced had changed her immunology, the gray matter in her brain, and reset her lifelong level of stress reactivity—making her a sitting duck for physical inflammation and autoimmune disease in adulthood, all surfacing at the very same age at which her own mother had died.

—

And how about Laura? Laura had an ACE Score of 4. According to the Adverse Childhood Experiences Study, Laura would get one score for each of the following emotional traumas of her youth: (1) an adult in her home routinely put her down and humiliated her; (2) she often felt that no one in her family loved her; (3) she often felt there was no one to protect her or look out for her; (4) Laura's parents divorced and a parent, her father, all but disappeared from her life.

Still, Laura at twenty seemed to be a bright young woman with a wonderful life ahead of her. You would never know that she was "shaking, invisibly, deep inside my cells," or that by the time she hit her mid-forties, she'd be suffering from early onset heart disease.

Indeed, even Laura is surprised that this cutting-edge research into the link between Adverse Childhood Experiences and adult well-being sheds new light on her adult health struggles. "I've never labeled my childhood as one full of adversity," Laura says. "It just was what it was. I'm not the only person who witnessed my parents' fights or had to go through their divorce, or who had to survive a lot of criticism from a parent struggling with a mental health issue. I muddled through, got out, and got on with my life. Isn't that what we all do?"

Still, she concedes, "I've often wondered what's wrong with me. Why does a confrontation with a client or a misunderstanding with my husband push me into a state of anxiety and dread for hours? Why are my anxiety sensors always going full blast? Why am I forty-six years old with heart disease and a defibrillator in my chest?" The research helps Laura to complete a puzzle.

John's ACE Score would be 3: a parent often put him down; he witnessed his mother being harmed; and, clearly, his father suffered from an undiagnosed behavioral health disorder, perhaps narcissism or depression, or both.

Georgia had an ACE Score of 3 as well.

Kat, Laura, John, and Georgia are hardly alone. Two-thirds of

American adults are carrying wounds from childhood quietly into adulthood, with little or no idea of how their wounds affect their daily health and well-being.

Something that happened to you when you were five or fifteen can land you in the hospital thirty years later, whether that something was headline news, or happened quietly, without anyone else knowing it, in the living room of your childhood home.

The New Theory of Everything

Scientists are calling the correlation between childhood trauma, brain architecture, and adult well-being the new psychobiological "theory of everything." Every few decades a groundbreaking psychosocial "theory of everything" helps us to develop a new playbook of understanding about why we are the way we are—and how we got that way. In the early twentieth century, Freudian psychoanalytic theory argued that the unconscious rules much of our waking life and dreams, and gave birth to the concept of the ego. Jungian theory taught, among other ideas, that we tend toward introversion or extroversion—leading Briggs and Myers to develop a personality indicator. More recently, neuroscientists discovered that "zero to three" was a critical synaptic window for brain development, giving birth to Head Start and preschool.

Today's understanding of Adverse Childhood Experiences revolutionizes how we see ourselves, our understanding of how we came to be the way we are, why we love the way we do, how we can better nurture our children, and how we can work to realize our potential.

Adverse Childhood Experience research shows that both physical and emotional suffering are rooted in the complex workings of the human immune system. The immune system is the body's master operating control center. What happens to the brain in childhood sets up the lifelong programming for this master operating system, governing all: body, brain, and mind.

The unifying principle of this new "theory of everything" is this: your emotional biography becomes your physical biology. And together they write much of the script for how you will live your life.

Put another way: your early stories script your biology and your biology scripts the way your life will play out.

Even "Mild" Childhood Adversity Matters

The adversity a child faces doesn't have to be severe abuse in order to create deep, biophysical changes that lead to chronic health conditions in adulthood.

"Our findings showed that the ten different types of adversity we examined were almost equal in their damage," says Felitti. After analyzing more than eighteen thousand responses, he and Anda found that no single Adverse Childhood Experience significantly trumped another. This was true even though some types, such as being sexually abused, are far worse in that society regards them as particularly shameful, and others such as physical abuse, are more overt in their violence. Interestingly, recurrent humiliation by a parent caused a slightly more detrimental impact and was marginally correlated to a greater likelihood of adult illness and depression. Simply living with a parent who puts you down and humiliates you, or who is alcoholic or depressed, can leave you with a profoundly hurtful ACE footprint and alter your brain and immunologic functioning for life.

According to Anda, the ACE Survey identifies only "the tip of the iceberg."

Other researchers agree. Over the past several years, scientists have been looking for ways to screen for types of childhood stressors that aren't included in the ACE Study. For instance, in 2014, researchers at the University of Cambridge asked parents of fourteen-year-olds to recall any negative life events or difficulties that their children—or that they as a family—had experienced between birth and the age of eleven. They asked questions about "family-focused" problems—including significant arguments or tension between parents, or simply lack of affection or communication between family members.

Brain imaging of these same kids when they were ages seventeen, eighteen, and nineteen found that even exposure to very common but relatively chronic forms of family dysfunction, such as lack of familial affection or parental discord, led to changes in the developing brain, decreasing the brain's size and volume.

The Childhood Trauma Questionnaire, or CTQ, is used with individuals ages twelve and older to screen for the lingering, invisible impact of more subtle forms of childhood hurt or neglect. The CTQ asks subtle questions such as, it was "never," "rarely," "sometimes," "often," or "very often" true that "People in my family said hurtful and insulting things to me," or that "People in my family called me things like 'stupid,' 'lazy,' or 'ugly.'"

The CTQ also screens for negative answers to positive statements, allowing a respondent to say that it was "rarely true" that "my family was a source of strength and support," or it was only "sometimes true" that "I felt loved." Because the CTQ lets respondents paint a more nuanced picture of their emotional experiences as children, it, too, has allowed researchers to demonstrate the striking scientific relationship between low-dose parental or family unkindness or neglect, damage to the young brain, and later negative health outcomes.

Chronic parental discord; enduring low-dose humiliation or blame and shame; chronic teasing; the quiet divorce between two secretly seething parents; a parent's premature exit from a child's life; the emotional scars of growing up with a hypercritical, unsteady, narcissistic, bipolar, alcoholic, addicted, or depressed parent; physical or emotional abuse or neglect: these happen in all too many families. Increasingly, it's understood that nonfamily stressors in childhood also can affect adult health. These include early medical trauma, being bullied or hazed, and living amid neighborhood violence. Although the details of individual experiences of adversity differ from one home to another and from one neighborhood to another, they are all precursors to the same organic chemical changes deep in the gray matter of the developing brain.

As Felitti observes, the years of "infancy and childhood are not lost, but, like a child's footprints in wet cement, lifelong." Or, as T. S. Eliot wrote in *Four Quartets*, "In my beginning is my end."

—

Of course, even though these positive correlations exist between early trauma and later illness, Adverse Childhood Experiences are not the sole contributor to adult disease. Disease develops for many reasons, including lifestyle, genetics, environmental toxins, and diet. We are not ill in adulthood simply because of what happened in our childhood. And we do not heal simply by knowing that childhood trauma and adversity play a role in adult illness.

But Felitti and Anda's research tells us that healing is more difficult if we do not recognize that our childhood plays a strong hand in whatever health problems we face now.

This is precisely why, today, in labs across the country, neuroscientists are peering into the once inscrutable brain-body connection, and breaking down, on a biochemical level, exactly how the early stress we face when we are very young, or teenagers, catches up with us when we are adults, altering our bodies, our cells, and even our DNA.

CHAPTER TWO

Different Adversities Lead to Similar Health Problems

The opening line of Tolstoy's *Anna Karenina*—"Happy families are all alike; every unhappy family is unhappy in its own way."—has inspired a philosophical dictum called "The Anna Karenina Principle." The idea is this: it's possible to fail at something in many ways; it's far harder to succeed at something—because success requires not failing in any of those ways.

Happy families may succeed not because of what they do right, but because of everything they don't do wrong. And according to ACE research, 64 percent of us grew up in families in which at least one thing went wrong: we've had at least one Adverse Childhood Experience. Every one of these unhappy families may be unhappy in its own, unique way. But there is one way in which unhappy families are alike, according to neurobiologists who study childhood adversity. Children from unhappy, dysfunctional families who experience chronic adversity undergo changes in brain architecture that create lasting physical scars that look pretty similar no matter who you are, where you lived, or what happened to make you unhappy when you were growing up.

How Your Biography Becomes Your Biology

To better understand how toxic childhood stress changes our brain, let's first review how our stress response is supposed to work when it's functioning optimally.

Let's say you're lying in bed and everyone else in the house is asleep. It's one a.m. You hear a creak on the steps. Then another creak. Now it sounds as if someone is in the hallway. You feel a sudden rush of alertness—even before your conscious mind weighs the possibilities of what might be going on. A small region in your brain known as the hypothalamus releases hormones that stimulate two little glands—the pituitary and adrenal glands—to pump chemicals throughout your body. Adrenaline and cortisol trigger immune cells to secrete powerful messenger molecules that whip up your body's immune response. Your pulse drums under your skin as you lie there, listening. The hair on the surface of your arms stands up. Muscles tighten. Your body gets charged up to do battle in order to protect life and limb.

Then you recognize those footsteps as those of your teenager coming up the steps after finishing his midnight bowl of cereal. Your body relaxes. Your muscles loosen. The hair on your arms flattens back down. Your hypothalamus, as well as your pituitary and adrenal glands—the "HPA stress axis"—calm down. And, whew, so do you.

When you have a healthy stress response, you respond quickly and appropriately to stress. After the stressful event, your body dampens down the fight-or-flight response. Your system recovers and returns to a baseline state of rest and recovery. In other words, you pass through both the first and the second half of the human stress cycle, coming full circle.

Even so, emotions affect our body in real and significant ways. Emotions are physical. We feel a "knot in our stomach," or get "all choked up," or see a relative or coworker as a "big pain in the neck."

There is a powerful relationship between mental stress and physical inflammation. When we experience stressful emotions—anger, fear, worry, anxiety, rumination, grief, loss—the HPA axis releases stress hormones, including cortisol and inflammatory cytokines, that promote inflammation.

Let's say your immune system has to fight a viral or bacterial infection. Lots of white blood cells charge to the site of the infection. Those white blood cells secrete inflammatory cytokines to help destroy the infiltrating pathogens and repair damaged tissues. However, when those cytokines aren't well regulated, or become too great in number, rather than repair tissue, they cause tissue damage. Toxic shock syndrome is an extreme example of how this can happen in the body very quickly.

More subtle types of tissue damage can happen slowly, over time, in response to chronic stress. When your system is repeatedly overstimulated, it begins to downshift its response to stress. On the face of it, that might sound like it's a good thing—as if a downshifted stress response should translate into less inflammation, right?

But remember, this stress response is supposed to react to a big stressor, pump into defensive action, then quickly recover and return to a state of quiet homeostasis, relaxing into rest and recovery. The problem is, when you are facing a lot of chronic stress, the stress response never shuts off. You're caught, perpetually, in the first half of the stress cycle. There is no state of recovery. Instead, the stress response is always mildly on—pumping out a chronic low dose of inflammatory chemicals. The stress glands—the hypothalamus, the HPA axis—secrete low levels of stress hormones all the time, leading to chronic cytokine activity and inflammation.

In simplest terms: chronic stress leads to a dysregulation of our stress hormones—which leads to unregulated inflammation. And inflammation translates into symptoms and disease.

This is the basic science on how stress hormones play a part in orchestrating our immune function and the inflammatory process. And it explains why we see such a significant link between individuals who experience chronic stress and significantly higher levels of inflammation and disease.

As Stanford professor Robert Sapolsky, PhD, a MacArthur Fellowship recipient for his research on the neurobiological impact of emotional stress on the immune system, has said, "The stress response does more damage than the stressor itself as we wallow in stress hormones."

Research bears out the relationship between stress and physical inflammation. For example, adults under the stress of taking care of spouses with dementia display increased levels of a cytokine that increases inflammation. Likewise, if an adult sibling dies, your risk of having a heart attack rises greatly. If you're pregnant and face a big, stressful event, your chance of miscarrying doubles. Encountering serious financial problems raises a man's risk of falling down and being injured in the months that follow. A child's death triples a parent's chance of developing multiple sclerosis. States of intense emotional fear or loss can precipitate a type of cardiomyopathy known as "broken heart syndrome," a severe physical weakening of the heart muscle that presents almost exactly like, and is often misdiagnosed as, a full-blown heart attack.

Why Stress Is More Damaging to a Child

Emotional stress in adult life affects us on a physical level in quantifiable, life-altering ways. But when children or teens meet up with emotional stressors and adversity, they leave even deeper scars. These potential stressors include chronic put-downs, emotional neglect, parental divorce, a parent's death, the mood shifts of a depressed or addicted parent, sexual abuse, medical trauma, the loss of a sibling, and physical or community violence. In each case, the HPA (hypothalamus-pituitary-adrenal) stress response can become reprogrammed so that it revs up one's inflammatory stress hormone response for the rest of one's life.

In young and growing children, the HPA stress axis is developing—and healthy maturation is heavily influenced by the safety or lack of safety we encounter in the day-to-day environment. When a young brain is repeatedly thrust into a state of hyperarousal or anxiety because of what's happening at a child's home, community, or school, the stress axis gets tipped into reaction over and over again, and the body becomes routinely flooded with inflammatory stress neurochemicals. This can lead to deep physiological changes that lead to long-lasting inflammation and disease.

—

More than half of women suffering from irritable bowel syndrome report childhood trauma. Children whose parents divorce are far more likely to have strokes as adults. ACE Scores are linked to a far greater likelihood of diseases including cancer, lung disease, diabetes, asthma, headaches, ulcers, multiple sclerosis, lupus, irritable bowel syndrome, and chronic fatigue.

The more categories of Adverse Childhood Experiences a child has faced, the greater the chances of developing heart disease as an adult. Again, a child who has 7 or more ACEs grows up with a 360 percent higher chance of developing heart disease.

Remember Laura? It's almost as if Laura had been living with a slow-brew version of broken heart syndrome. Eventually, the emotional loss of never having had a reliable parent was manifested in her own adult heart.

Medical Adverse Experience

Not all Adverse Childhood Experiences are about poor parenting.

Michele had the kind of lovely parents who created a home life that fits the happy family mold; they gave their son and daughter all the parental love and support that every child deserves. "Life was good," Michele says. Then, when she was thirteen years old, she had a bladder infection and was placed on a routine course of antibiotics. "Within twenty-four hours I had a headache and rash."

Michele's doctor told Michele's mom, "it's a virus."

But the rash didn't go away. Michele started wincing at bright lights. The eye doctor couldn't figure out what was wrong. Blisters began developing along her upper lip. The pediatrician didn't know what to do, so Michele's parents took her to the hospital. They saw a dermatologist who had read about Michele's symptoms in an article. He thought she might have Stevens-Johnson syndrome, or SJS, a rare illness caused by a severe allergic reaction to a medication.

Michele was admitted to Columbia-Presbyterian hospital in New York City. Within twenty-four hours blisters the size of large hands broke out across her body. At first, they covered "30 percent of my body, then 100 percent," Michele says. She was diagnosed with an advanced form of SJS, known as toxic epidermal necrolysis syndrome, or TENS. The bowl-sized blisters began to "connect and combine until my entire torso was one enormous blister. Even my corneas were blistered."

Today, when patients develop TENS, they're put in an induced coma, because the physical pain is simply too unbearable. But in 1981, when Michele was diagnosed with the illness, doctors "just watched the progression." Her physicians converted Michele's hospital room into a burn unit—she looked like a burn victim, so she was treated as if she'd been rescued from a fire. "I felt as if I were being scalped over every inch of my skin." Michele says she started dissociating from her body. "My body and I parted ways in that hospital, we stopped talking to each other. I couldn't bear to feel that pain."

Miraculously, Michele survived. She missed two months of school, while her mom helped to nurse her back to health. Little by little, life began to regain a rhythm of normality—except for the fear Michele still carried within. Every year on the anniversary of the day she was first admitted to the hospital, "my hair would fall out," she says. "Then it would grow slowly back in." Michele attended the University of Pennsylvania and held it together, but the whole time, she says, "I was having insomnia and recurring nightmares." In her late twenties she was diagnosed with chronic fatigue, Epstein-Barr virus, and irritable bowel syndrome. "I had terrible muscle pains all over my body and chronic sinus infections. I had trouble sitting still for even five minutes because of the pain." Her liver enzymes went "sky high." It was, she says, "one mysterious illness after another."

And then, at the age of thirty-five, Michele's doctor sat her down and told her that she had "severe, advanced osteoporosis." Her bones were going to start disintegrating, he said. "If we don't get this under control, sometime in the next ten years your bones are going to spontaneously crumble."

Michele's early adversity had nothing to do with bad parenting. But her early life stress was extreme, and the damage that stress did to her developing immune system and cells was just as corrosive.

———

Life is complex and messy, and suffering comes in many forms. Bad things happen. Parents get sick or pass away. Accidents come out of nowhere, as do medical crises.

How do the biophysical changes and inflammation triggered by very different types of early childhood adversity translate years later into autoimmune diseases, heart disease, and cancer?

Flipping Crucial Genetic Switches

On an unusually brisk December morning, Margaret McCarthy, PhD, professor of neuroscience at the University of Maryland School of Medicine, meets me at a downtown Baltimore coffee shop. Her schedule is tight, so we pick up two cups of soup to go and head to her office.

As we enter the hall that serves as the main artery for McCarthy's four-room lab, we pass a sign that says, "Research saves lives," on a large photo of a young, smiling girl holding a stuffed bunny. McCarthy has taught science for years to med students, grad students, and even high schoolers—whom she takes on as lab assistants to help "turn them on to science."

She offers a primer on what research has unveiled about childhood adversity and altered brain development.

"Early stress causes changes in the brain that reset the immune system so that either you no longer respond to stress or you respond in an exacerbated way and can't shut off that stress response," she says.

This change to our lifelong stress response happens through a process known as epigenetics. Epigenetic changes occur when early environmental influences both good (nurturing caregivers, a healthy diet, clean air and water) and bad (stressful conditions, poor diet, infections, or harmful chemicals) permanently alter which genes become active in the body.

These epigenetic shifts take place due to a process called gene methylation. McCarthy explains, "Our DNA is not just sitting there. It's wrapped up very tightly and coated in protected proteins, which together make up the chromosome. It doesn't matter what your genome is; what matters is how your genome is expressed. And for genes to be expressed properly, the chromosome has to be unwound and opened up, like a flower, right at that particular gene."

McCarthy unfurls the fingers of both hands. "Imagine this," she says. "You're watching a flower bloom, and as it opens up, it's covered with blemishes." She folds several of her fingers back in, as if they're suddenly unable to budge. "Those blemishes keep it from flourishing as it otherwise would. If, when our DNA opens up, it's covered with these methylation marks, that gene can't express itself properly in the way that it should."

When such "epigenetic silencing" occurs, McCarthy continues, these small chemical markers—also known as methyl groups—adhere to specific genes that are supposed to govern the activity of stress hormone receptors in our brain. These chemical markers silence important genes in the segment of our genome that oversees our hippocampus's regulation of stress hormones in adulthood. When the brain can't moderate our biological stress response, it goes into a state of constant hyperarousal and reactivity. Inflammatory hormones and chemicals keep coursing through the body at the slightest provocation.

In other words, when a child is young and his brain is still developing, if he is repeatedly thrust into a state of fight or flight, this chronic stress state causes these small, chemical markers to disable the genes that regulate the stress response—preventing the brain from properly regulating its response for the rest of his life.

Researcher Joan Kaufman, PhD, director of the Child and Adolescent Research and Education (CARE) program at Yale School of Medicine, analyzed the DNA in the saliva of ninety-six children who'd been taken away from their parents due to abuse or neglect as well as that of ninety-six other children who were living in what we might think of as seemingly happy family settings. Kaufman found significant differences in epigenetic markers in the DNA of the children who'd faced hardship—in almost three thousand sites on their DNA, and on all twenty-three chromosomes.

The children who'd been maltreated and separated from their parents showed epigenetic changes in specific sites on the human genome that determine how appropriately and effectively they will later respond to life's stressors.

Seth Pollak, PhD, professor of psychology and director of the Child Emotion Laboratory at the University of Wisconsin, found that fifty children with a history of adversity and trauma showed changes in a gene that helps to manage stress by signaling the cortisol response to quiet down so that the body can return to a calm state after a stressor. But because this gene was damaged, the body couldn't rein in its heightened stress response. Says Pollak, "A crucial set of brakes are off."

This is only one of hundreds of genes that are altered when a child faces adversity.

When the HPA stress axis is overloaded in childhood or the teenage years, it leads to long-lasting side effects—not just because of the impact stress has on us at that time in our lives, but also because early chronic stress biologically reprograms how we will react to stressful events for our entire lives. That long-term change creates a new physiological set point for how actively our endocrine and immune function will churn out a damaging cocktail of stress neurochemicals that barrage our bodies and cells when we're thirty, forty, fifty, and beyond. Once the stress system is damaged, we overrespond to stress and our ability to recover naturally from that reactive response mode is impaired. We're always responding.

Imagine for a moment that your body receives its stress hormones and chemicals through an IV drip that's turned on high when needed, and when the crisis passes, it's switched off again. Now think of it this way: kids whose brains have undergone epigenetic changes because of early adversity have an inflammation-promoting drip of fight-or-flight hormones turned on high every day—and there is no off switch.

When the HPA stress system is turned on and revved to go all the time, we are always caught in that first half of the stress cycle. We unwittingly marinate in those inflammatory chemicals for decades, which sets the stage for symptoms to be at full throttle years down the road—in the form of irritable bowel syndrome, autoimmune disease, fibromyalgia, chronic fatigue, fibroid tumors, ulcers, heart disease, migraines, asthma, and cancer.

These changes that make us vulnerable to specific diseases are already evident *in* childhood. Joan Kaufman and her colleagues discovered, in the first study to find such direct correlations, that children who had been neglected showed significant epigenetic differences "across the entire genome" including in genes implicated in cardiovascular disease, diabetes, obesity, and cancer.

Yet by the time signs of an autoimmune condition creep up at forty or a heart condition rears its head at fifty, we often can't link what happened when we were children to our adult illness. We become used to that old sense of emotional stress, of not being okay. It just seems normal. We have a long daily commute, a thirty-year mortgage, and our particular mix of family dynamics. We generally deal and we're usually okay. Then something minuscule happens: we have an argument with our sister over something said at a family dinner; we get a notice in the mail that our insurance isn't going to cover a whopping medical bill; the refrigerator tanks the day before a big dinner party; our boss approves a colleague's ideas in a meeting and ignores ours; a car honks long and hard as it swerves from behind to cut in front of us on the freeway. We react to these events as if they are a matter of life or death. We trigger easily. We begin to realize that we're not so fine.

An adult who came of age without experiencing traumatic childhood stress might meet the same stressor and experience that same spike in cortisol, but once that stressor has passed, he or she quickly returns to a state of rest and relaxation. But if we had early trauma, our adult HPA stress axis can't distinguish between real danger and perceived stress. Each time we get sidetracked by a stressful event, it sends split-second signals that cause our immune system to rev into high gear. We get that adrenaline rush but the genes that should tell our stress system to return to a state of rest and relaxation don't do their job.

Over days and years, the disparity between a long "cortisol recovery" period and a short one makes a significant, life-changing difference in the number of hours we spend marinating in our own inflammatory stress hormones. And over time, that can deeply distort your life.

The Ever-Alert Child

Adults with Adverse Childhood Experiences are on alert. It's a habit they learned in childhood, when they couldn't be sure when they'd face the next high-tension situation.

After her terrifying childhood illness, Michele never felt at peace, or whole, as an adult: "I was afraid I could be blindsided by any small medical crisis that could morph and change my entire life."

Laura, as an adult, holds a high-profile DC job that requires lightning decisions and heightened awareness. She's good at it since, as a child, Laura and her brain learned to always be on high alert for the next snipe from her mother, as if being prepared could make it hurt less. "I became an expert at gauging my mom's moods," she says. "Whenever I was in the same room with her, I was thinking about how to slink away."

By the time she was nine, Laura had learned to be "unconsciously on the lookout for a very subtle narrowing of my mom's eyes," which would tell her that she was about to be blamed for "something I didn't even know that I'd done—like eating half of a sandwich in the fridge or taking too long to tie my shoe." Laura grew up "learning to toe my way forward, as if blindfolded, to figure out what was coming next, where the next emotional ledge might be, so I wouldn't get too near to my mother's sharp edges."

From Laura's perspective, her mom was dangerous. "I knew she would never physically hurt me," she explains. "But I was terrified—even when she was in a good mood. At night, when I would hear her lightly snoring, I would feel this overwhelming sense of freedom, relief."

Laura's life was never at risk of course—she lived in a safe suburban neighborhood, had food to eat, clothes to wear. But she felt as if her life was at stake. Like all children whose parents display terrifying behavior, Laura carried the overwhelming biological fear that if her primary caregiver turned against her, she would not survive. After all, if the person upon whom you depend for food, shelter, and life itself, turns on you, how are you going to stay alive in the world? You feel as if your life depends on the adult's goodwill, because when you were very small, how your caregiver treated you really was a matter of life or death.

As an adult, Laura "schooled" herself to believe that the early adversity she faced wasn't that bad compared with that of other people who also grew up with alcoholic, angry, divorced, or depressed parents. She keeps telling herself that she's over her childhood troubles.

But her body is far from over them. Laura lives with heart disease and a defibrillator in her chest. Like Michele, her anxiety sensors are set on high alert, and she doesn't know how to turn them off.

The Rattled Cage

We might reasonably intuit that some types of childhood adversity are more damaging to us than others. For instance, we'd expect that the trauma that Kat experienced in knowing that her father murdered her mother would have a dramatically worse biological impact on her than Laura's having been chronically put down by her depressive mom.

We'd certainly assume that Kat's story would be more biologically damaging than that of Ellie, who was the second youngest of five children and grew up in a quiet suburban neighborhood outside Philadelphia. Ellie remembers having a very close relationship with her parents, but, as she got older, she says, "I knew something wasn't right. My two oldest brothers were time bombs of violent emotion, just waiting to go off. Sitting at the dinner table with my parents, talking about politics, they'd start fighting each other over nothing at all—and the fights got ugly."

Soon the boys were getting into trouble with alcohol and drugs— "and the police started showing up." Ellie recalls, "I'd often hear my parents and my brothers screaming at each other at two in the morning.

My mom and dad would come in my room and tell my little sister and me not to be scared, that everything was okay, but it was terrifying," especially when her older brother ended up in jail.

Ellie got good grades, despite the stressors at home, and went to college in California on an athletic scholarship. But, after college, she began having suicidal thoughts and, at age twenty-four, was diagnosed with severe autoimmune psoriasis. "My body was attacking itself," she says.

According to ACE research, growing up with a family member who is in jail is related to a much higher risk of poor health-related outcomes as an adult.

Laura, John, Georgia, Kat, Michele, and Ellie tell six unique stories of childhood adversity. And yet their brains reacted to these different levels of trauma in a similar biological way. The developing brain reacts to different types and degrees of trauma so similarly because all the categories of Adverse Childhood Experience stressors have a very simple common denominator: they are all unpredictable. The child can't predict exactly when, why, or from where the next emotional or physical hit is coming.

Researchers refer to stress that happens in unpredictable ways and at unpredictable times as "chronic unpredictable stress," and they have been studying its effects on animal development for decades—long before Felitti and Anda's investigation into ACEs first began. In classic studies, investigators expose animals to different types of stressors for several weeks, to see how those stressful stimuli affect their behavior. In one experiment, McCarthy and her postdocs exposed male and female rats to three weeks of chronic unpredictable mild stress. Every day, rats were exposed to a few low-grade stressors: their cage was rotated; they were given a five-minute swim, their bedding was dampened; they went for a day without food; they were physically restrained for thirty minutes; or they were exposed to thirty minutes of strobe lights.

At the end of the three weeks, McCarthy's team examined the rats to evaluate brain differences. In the group exposed to chronic unpredictable mild stress, she and her team found significant changes in the receptors in the brain's hippocampus—an area of the brain associated with emotion, which would normally help modulate stress hormone production and put the brakes on feelings of stress and anxiety after a stressor has passed.

The rats who'd been exposed to chronic unpredictable stress weren't able to turn off the stress response, but the control group that experienced no stress showed no brain changes.

However, when stress is completely predictable, even if it is more traumatic—such as giving a rat a regularly scheduled foot shock accompanied by a sharp, loud sound—the stress does not create these exact same brain changes. "Rats exposed to a much more traumatic stressor get used to it if it happens at the same time and in the same way every day," says McCarthy. "They manage. They know it's coming, then it's over." Moreover, she says, "They don't show signs of these same brain changes, or inflammation, or illness."

On the other hand, she adds, "if you introduce more moderate but unpredictable stressful experiences at a different time each day, with different levels of intensity, adding in different noises, such as loud clapping at unpredictable intervals, those rats show significant changes to the brain. And they get physically sick; they get ulcers."

This is why researchers believe that it is the unpredictability of stress that is particularly damaging. On a walking tour of her lab, McCarthy points out the metal stand on which rodents' cages can be gently shaken for a short time. "Even the most mild unpredictable stressors, something as simple as gently shaking the cage, playing rock music, putting a new object in the cage that they aren't used to, all these cause very specific changes in the brain when we do them without warning."

The bottom line, McCarthy says, is that the brain can "tolerate severely stressful events if they are predictable, but you cannot tolerate even mild stressful events if they are very unpredictable."

Yet even though researchers have known for years about the effects of chronic unpredictable stress on the adult brain, only recently have they examined what happens to the brains of children exposed to chronic unpredictable stressors.

The Difficulty of Not Knowing

Mary, now in her midfifties, grew up as the oldest of four kids in a small town in Oregon. Life with her artist parents was a lot like living with unpredictable cage rattling, shaking, and odd, loud noises. Mary's dad had his own damaged childhood. He'd grown up never knowing who his own dad was, and his mom died when he was seven. His maternal grandparents adopted his brother, but not him because his parents hadn't married, and he was seen as damaged goods. (His ACE Score was very high.)

Years later, when he was a father of four, he drank heavily, partied, and played cards. "I remember hearing my dad and friends, up all night drinking and swearing really loud in the living room outside my bedroom, even on school nights. I didn't feel safe." Mary has large, sympathetic eyes and shoulder-length brown hair that she neatly tucks behind her ears with long, graceful fingers. "I can remember my mother yelling at him, 'You need to make them leave. Your children can't sleep!' And he'd yell back, 'I can't make them leave, these are my friends!' My sleep—and sense of being safe—weren't important to him."

Mary's mother was managing her own anxiety that came with having four children and being stuck in a marriage with an alcoholic, so she, too, was emotionally absent. "I got bullied a lot in grade school," Mary tells me. "I was scrawny and short and kids would terrorize me." Her mom was preoccupied with an affair her dad was having and didn't listen to Mary's problems; eventually she took Mary and her younger siblings to the East Coast to live with her own mother.

"A part of me quite enjoyed that time away from all the partying and the tension in their marriage, the fighting," says Mary.

After her parents got back together, at first Mary was happy and hopeful. But her dad was still drinking heavily. He'd get so drunk that "my mom would literally kick him out of bed and he'd come sleep with me." Nothing happened, Mary says, "nothing like that." But still, it was disconcerting to sometimes wake in the night at age ten to find her dad in bed with her, sleeping off another drunken stupor.

At school things hadn't improved much. "We were still wearing dresses back then," says Mary. "All the boys called me 'Gladiator' because when they'd tease me I'd go at them, I'd fight back." That made the bullying worse. "They'd chase me and hold me down on the ground and forcibly pull off my underwear."

Mary didn't even think of telling her father about the bullying. "When he was drunk, he would spank us really hard. Once when my sister was in second grade, he pulled down her pants and spanked her in front of all his drunken friends."

Mary's sensors were always on high alert—getting ready for the next unpredictable, incoming emotional bomb. Her stress axis was constantly kicking into high gear; her immune system, in overdrive. By then, Mary had started to show signs of an autoimmune disorder called vitiligo, in which the body's immune cells attack the pigmentation in the skin. Areas of her skin turned white, as if the skin had been bleached or burned in the past and new skin was trying to form over it.

"Our skin is our first line of defense against the world, the thing that's supposed to keep us safe, secure our physical boundaries," Mary says. "And yet my parents hadn't set any boundaries to keep me or my siblings safe." It was as if her skin were pleading for her parents to set those boundaries—the kind of safe zone parents are supposed to set for kids.

Even worse than the skin disorder, however, "were my constant stomachaches," she recalls. "I'd have chronic constipation and cramping, and then terrible diarrhea—all the symptoms of irritable bowel, though we didn't know what to call it back then." Sometimes, she'd find herself getting physically jittery and nervous "seemingly for no reason. I'd just be standing there and I'd get these rushes of fear, ripping and prickling through my body."

Over time, her father's boundaryless behavior grew more bizarre. When Mary was fourteen, he cut out hundreds of naked bodies from a stack of old *Playboys*, took off their heads, and pasted their disembodied boobs, legs, butts, and crotches on the walls of the kitchen. Andrea, one of Mary's few friends, told her parents about the "wallpaper." "After that, Andrea wasn't allowed at my house," Mary says. "I started to realize that other kids weren't comfortable around me because of my dad."

When she was fifteen, her parents moved to a house in the country. "I think they were trying to salvage their marriage." One crisp winter night, when Mary was coming out of the garage, one of her dad's drunken friends was standing by his car in the driveway. "As I walked by to go in the house he stared at me hard and said, 'You are so beautiful!' Then he threw me into the backseat of his car and got on top of me. He stuck his tongue down my throat and was groping me."

Mary forced him off and ran in to tell her dad, who was also drunk. "He told me to stop making such a big deal about it."

And yet, at other times, Mary's dad did show concern for her. Once, when Mary was in a car accident, "he got in the ambulance with me and cried the whole way to the hospital." He was completely unpredictable.

By the time she was eighteen, Mary had developed "unwavering depression," which would progress over the next thirty years—getting worse after she married and had her four children. She developed a severe lower back problem that worsened every year. And her autoimmune vitiligo started to cover her arms and neck.

"I fell into a postpartum depression after each birth, and after my fourth son, I was suicidal. My physical and emotional pain had snow-balled. If I was driving without any of my kids in the car, I'd find myself thinking, 'How can I crash this car into a tree in such a way that no one will know it's suicide, and so that I'm not just impaired and a burden to my family afterward?' "

And that was when, says Mary, "I realized something potent was haunting me; something was terribly wrong with how unsafe I felt in the world. I had these beautiful sons and I just didn't feel okay inside in any way, shape, or form."

—

To the developing brain, knowing what's coming next matters most. This makes sense if you think back to how the stress response works optimally. You meet a bear in the woods and your body floods with adrenaline and cortisol so that you can decide quickly: do you run away or try to frighten away the bear? After you deal with the crisis, you recover, your stress hormones abate, and you go home with a great story.

McCarthy presents another situation. "What if that bear is circling the house and you can't get away from it and you never know if it's going to strike, or when, or what it will do next? There it is, threatening you every single day. You can't fight or flee." Then, she says, "Your emergency response system is set into overdrive over and over again. Your anxiety sensors are always going full blast."

Even subtle, common forms of childhood stress—e.g., a hypercritical, narcissistic, or manic-depressive parent—can cause just as much damage as a parent who deals out angry, physical beatings or just disappears.

And in that sense, Kat's story and Mary's story are very similar to Laura's, John's, Georgia's, Michele's, and Ellie's. All of them, even in adult life, felt that the bear was still out there, somewhere, circling in the woods, stalking, and might strike again any day, anytime.

—

According to Vincent Felitti, the one area in which a "yes" answer on the Adverse Childhood Experiences questionnaire has been correlated to a slightly higher level of adult negative health outcomes is in response to ACE question number 1, which addresses the issue of "chronic humiliation." Would adults in the home often swear at you, insult you, put you down, or humiliate you?

This strong correlation between adverse health problems and unpredictable, chronic humiliation by a parent suggests that it is not knowing if you are safe from the "bear" that matters most.

There are a lot of bears out there. Depression, bipolar disease, alcohol, and other addictions are remarkably prevalent adult afflictions. According to the National Institute of Mental Health, over 18 percent of adults, or nearly forty-four million Americans, suffer from a diagnosable mental health disorder in any given year. Twenty-three million adult Americans suffer from an alcohol or drug addiction. Indeed, according to the original ACE Study, one in four people with Adverse Childhood Experiences had a parent who was addicted to alcohol.

Often, alcoholism and depression go hand in hand—addiction can be an unconscious effort to self-medicate a mood disorder. But even when they are not working in tandem, mood disorders and alcoholism share one thing: both make adults behave in emotionally undependable ways. The parent who hugs you one day when picking you up from school might humiliate you in front of your friends the next afternoon. The sense of not knowing what's coming next never goes away.

The Sadness Seed

Adversity in childhood can be the precursor to deep depression and anxiety later in life. A growing body of research shows that there is a close correlation between Adverse Childhood Experiences and emotional health disorders in adulthood. In Felitti and Anda's Adverse

Childhood Experiences Study, 18 percent of individuals with an ACE Score of 1 had suffered from clinical depression, and the likelihood rose sharply with each ACE Score. Thirty percent of those with an ACE Score of 3—and nearly 50 percent of those with an ACE Score of 4 or more—had suffered from chronic depression.

Twelve and a half percent of respondents to the Adverse Childhood Experiences Study cite having an ACE Score of 4 or more.

For women, the correlation is even more disturbing. While 19 percent of men with an ACE Score of 1 suffered from clinical depression, 24 percent of women with that score did. Likewise, while 24 percent of men with a score of 2 developed adult clinical depression, 35 percent of women did. Thirty percent of men with a score of 3 developed clinical depression, compared to 42 percent of women who had three categories of Adverse Childhood Experiences. And 35 percent of men, versus nearly 60 percent of women, with a score of 4 or more suffered from chronic depression.

The strongest precursor of adult depression turned out to be Adverse Childhood Experiences that fell into the category of "childhood emotional abuse."

Whether you are male or female, the loss of a parent in childhood triples your chances of depression in adulthood. Being raised by a mother who suffers from depression puts you at a higher risk of living with chronic pain as an adult. Children who experienced severe trauma before the age of sixteen are three times more likely to develop schizophrenia later in life.

Most disturbing are the statistics on suicide: while only 1 percent of those with an ACE Score of 0 have ever attempted suicide, almost one in five individuals with an ACE Score of 4 or more has tried to end his or her life. Indeed, a person with an ACE Score of 4 or more is, statistically, 1,220 percent more likely to attempt suicide than someone with an ACE Score of 0.

It certainly makes sense that childhood emotional trauma will spill out in our adulthood. Psychology and psychotherapy help us understand the link between our childhood wounds and adult emotional problems, and making this connection can help free us from the pain of our past.

But research tells us that often, childhood adversity leads to more deep-seated changes within the brain, and that depression and mood dysregulation are also set in motion on a cellular and neurobiological level.

So what is causing neurobiological changes inside the brain itself?

How Early Adversity Changes the Shape and Size of the Brain

When a young child faces emotional adversity or stressors, cells in the brain release a hormone that actually shrinks the size of the brain's developing hippocampus—altering his or her ability to process emotion and manage stress. Magnetic resonance imaging (MRI) studies show that the higher an individual's childhood trauma score, the smaller the cerebral gray matter, or brain volume, is in key processing areas of the brain, including the prefrontal cortex, an area related to decision-making and self-regulatory skills; the amygdala, or fear-processing center of the brain; and the sensory association cortices and cerebellum, both of which affect how we process and regulate emotions and moods.

MRIs also show that kids raised in orphanages have much smaller brains than those of others. That smaller brain volume may be due to a reduction in the brain's gray matter—which is made up of brain cells, or neurons—as well as white matter, which includes nerves (with coated, or myelinated, axons) that allow for the fast transmission of messages in the brain. Other studies show that this smaller-sized amygdala in adults who've experienced childhood maltreatment shows marked "hyperactivity." Frontal regions of the brain display "atypical activation" throughout daily life—making individuals hyperreactive to even very small stressors.

The Inflamed Brain

"Early stress impacts the developing brain in a way that, until very recently, we just didn't think was possible," McCarthy says. "It turns out that chronic, early unpredictable stress can trigger a process of low-grade inflammation within the brain itself."

That is pretty revolutionary news. Until recently, most scientists thought that inflammation could not be generated by the brain. "We thought that the brain was what we call 'immune-privileged,'" explains McCarthy. "Inflammation in the brain occurred only when there was an external event, such as a brain injury or head trauma, or an infection such as meningitis."

But, "That has turned out not to be the case. When we are chronically stressed, the brain responds by creating a state of neuroinflammation. And that neuroinflammation can be present at levels that, until very recently, we could not even detect."

This type of inflammation develops due to a type of non-neuronal brain cell known as microglia. Our microglial cells make up about one-tenth of our brain cells. For years, researchers thought that these microglia cells were "just there to get rid of stuff we didn't need," explains McCarthy. "They were taking out the trash, so to speak."

Microglia play an integral role in pruning our brain's neurons and in brain development. They are crucial to the normal processing of the brain all the time, continuously scanning their environment, determining, Are we good here? Or not so good? Are we safe? Or not safe?

Shake the cage. Flash the lights. The microglia in the brain take note, fast. They don't like chronic, unpredictable stress. They don't like it at all.

"Microglia go off kilter in the face of chronic unpredictable stress," says McCarthy. "They get really worked up, they crank out neurochemicals that lead to neuroinflammation. And this below-the-radar state of chronic neuroinflammation can lead to changes that reset the tone of the brain for life."

"It is very possible that when microglia go off kilter, they are actually pruning away neurons," McCarthy says. That is, they are killing off brain cells that we need.

In a healthy brain, microglia control the number of neurons that the cerebral cortex needs—but unhappy microglia can excessively prune away cells in areas that would normally play a key role in basic executive functions, like reasoning and impulse control. They are essential in a healthy brain, but in the face of chronic unpredictable stress, they can start eating away at the brain's synapses.

"In some cases, microglia are engulfing and destroying dying neurons, and they are taking out the trash, just as we always thought," says McCarthy. "But in other cases, microglia are destroying healthy neurons—and in that case, it's more like murder." This excessive pruning can lead to what McCarthy refers to as a "reset tone" in the brain. You might think of that stressed brain as a muscle that's lost its tone and is atrophying. And that loss of gray and white matter can trigger depression, anxiety disorders, and even more extreme psychopathology such as schizophrenia and Alzheimer's disease.

Microglia may also prune a special group of neurons in the hippocampus that are capable of regenerating. "We used to think that you could never make new neurons but one of the most revolutionary new findings in the last decade is the discovery that there are new neurons being born in the hippocampus all the time," says McCarthy. The growth of new neurons is very important to adult mental health. "If something interferes with their growth, depression can set in." Indeed research suggests, says McCarthy, that "microglia, when they are overly exuberant, may kill these new neurons as soon as they are born."

Scientists have introduced healthy microglia back into the mouse brain. The results have been stunning: once mice brains are repopulated with microglia, all signs of depression completely disappear.

So much depends on the microglia in our brain being happy, unrattled. So much depends on our microglia not pruning away too many neurons.

We might hypothesize that "angry, worked-up microglia could impair the growth of healthy new neurons in the brain's hippocampus," says McCarthy. "When healthy neurons in the hippocampus die, our emotional well-being would be impaired over the long term."

Facing situation after situation of sudden and unpredictable stress in childhood can trigger microglia to prune away important neurons and initiate a state of neuroinflammation that resets the tone of the brain, creating the conditions for long-lasting anxiety and depression.

A Perfect Storm: Childhood Stress, Brain Pruning, and Adolescence

When children come into adolescence, they naturally undergo a period of developmental pruning of neurons. When we are very young, we have an overproduction of neurons and synaptic connections. Some of them die off naturally to allow us to "turn down the noise in the brain," says McCarthy, and to increase our mastery in skills that interest us. The brain prepares for becoming more specialized at the things we're good at and interested in, while we lose what we don't need.

But if, due to childhood stress, lots of neurons and synapses have already been pruned away, then when the natural pruning that occurs during adolescence begins to take place, and the brain starts to naturally prune neurons it doesn't need so that a teenager can focus on building particular skills—baseball, singing, poetry—then, suddenly, there may be too much pruning going on.

Dan Siegel, MD, child neuropsychiatrist and clinical professor at the University of California, Los Angeles (UCLA), is the pioneer of a growing field known as "interpersonal biology," which integrates the fields of neuroscience and psychology. According to Siegel, "The stress of Adverse Childhood Experiences causes toxicity to the neurons and neural pathways that integrate different areas of the brain." When adolescent pruning occurs in the integrated circuitry between the hippocampus, which is important in storing memories; the corpus callosum, which links the left and right hemispheres of the brain; and the prefrontal cortex, these brain changes, says Siegel, have a profound effect on our decision-making abilities, self-regulatory processes, attention, emotional regulation, thoughts, and behavior.

When these integrated circuits are affected by adversity, or genetic vulnerability, or both, during preadolescence, says Siegel, and then puberty hits, "adolescent pruning pares down the existing but insufficient number of integrated fibers, which makes a child vulnerable to mood dysregulation. It is when this brain integration is impaired that a dysfunction in mood regulation may emerge."

Imagine, hypothetically speaking, that all kids start with 4,000 neurons (that's a made-up number, for illustration purposes). Now, let's say that we have two five-year-old boys, Sam and Joe. Sam faces early adversity and Joe doesn't. As Sam meets up with chronic unpredictable stress in his childhood, his neurons are slowly pruned away. By the time Sam is twelve, after a lot of stress-related neuronal pruning, he has 1,800 neurons left. He is still okay, functioning well; 1,800 neurons are enough (using our hypothetical numbers) to get by on, since kids start out with so many more than they need in the first place.

But then Sam and Joe both go through the adolescent period of neuronal pruning. Let's say that Sam and Joe, like all kids, each lose a hypothetical 1,000 more neurons during adolescence. Sam, who grew up with early chronic unpredictable stress, begins to emerge with a notably different brain from Joe.

Suddenly, the difference between Sam's brain and Joe's trauma-free brain becomes extreme. Joe, who's grown up fairly adversity free, still has his 3,000 neurons—plenty to go forward and live a healthy and happy life. Meanwhile, Sam is left with only 800 neurons.

And that makes all the difference. It is not enough for the brain to function in a healthy manner.

For kids who have already had pruning due to early stress, Siegel explains, "when average adolescent pruning occurs, what remains may be insufficient for mood to be kept in balance. If stressors are high, this pruning process may be even more intense, and more of the at-risk circuits may be diminished in number and effectiveness."

The child who faced Adverse Childhood Experiences will be more likely to develop depression, bipolar disorder, eating disorders, anxiety disorders, or poor executive function and decision making—many of which can lead to substance abuse. This may be why, statistically, so many young people first show signs of depression or bipolar disorders in high school, and in college—even kids who just a year or two earlier seemed absolutely fine.

—

Stephen's parents, both investment bankers, were hardly around when he was growing up in New York City. Stephen ate dinner at night with his older sister and their nanny. When his parents came home around nine o'clock, a time when most kids were getting tucked into bed and kissed good night, they'd all sit down together at the kitchen table, and the nanny would give her daily report. She was an older woman who loved to "give a laundry list of what we'd done wrong." Stephen "lived in fear of that moment. Especially for my sister."

His sister, who was five years older, was "already expected to be a genius like our parents, by the time she was in fourth grade. If she brought home an eighty-five on a math test, my parents would drill her on math problems until eleven o'clock." Then, they'd tell their friends at the next weekend party at our country house how "Alexis is already doing algebra!"

Stephen, as the baby, often got off lightly when he was young, and recalls feeling "that my parents loved me and wanted everything for me. But they were also terrifying."

As Stephen got older, his parents stopped "treating me like the cute baby." He did well academically and his standardized test scores were sometimes off the charts. "My parents decided that I must be the genius they'd been waiting for. I got their laser focus."

But he soon started to feel that "I wasn't as smart as my parents hoped I'd be." When he was nine, Stephen started having acute asthma attacks. He was also "perpetually forgetful. I'd lose everything. I'd forget to bring my sweater or my Spanish book home. I'd leave my clarinet in the band room. It made my parents furious. They'd tell me, 'Get it together! We don't have time for your nonsense, Stephen!'" Once, while staying at a plush lakeside resort, he walked into water with his flip-flops on to look for tadpoles. As he walked out, one flip-flop got stuck in the mud. "I tried to find it. I was digging in the muck. My dad just lost it. He stood on the edge of the lake yelling, 'You lost your flip-flop? Really, Stephen? You can't take a walk without losing your shoes? You think we're going to just buy you another pair? We're not buying you anything!'" On the ride home, Stephen had a full-blown asthma attack.

Stephen was also a "nonjock." He liked to read more than he liked to play ball. "My dad started calling me 'pretty boy.' I'd come in the door from being at a concert with my friends and he'd say, 'Hey, pretty boy, good time?' He was pissed that I hadn't spent the weekend on an athletic field the way he had when he was seventeen, the way his colleagues' and friends' kids were."

As many adult children recall, "it wasn't all bad. My dad taught me how to fish, how to sail, and how to analyze the financial pages of the newspaper. My mom left work to come to every single concert I was in when I played in the state youth orchestra. Sometimes when my dad was out of town, she'd let my sister and me snuggle in her bed and we'd watch movies and eat sandwiches from the deli downstairs. She'd tell me, 'Your dad loves you so much, he's just very stressed with work, it's not about you, Stevie.' She was not affectionate. But she tried."

In high school Stephen, despite high test scores, couldn't seem to manage his workload and get papers in on time, and was diagnosed with attention deficit disorder, high stakes performance anxiety—and depression. "I just stopped wanting to go out with my friends, or do anything. I wanted the world to just let me be." Then he developed a condition known as alopecia areata, in which the immune system attacks the hair follicles and segments of hair fall out, leaving bald patches. "My hair started falling out in huge chunks.'"

Stephen went on to grad school, getting his PhD in psychology. Today, Stephen is forty-two, a high school counselor. He shaves his head so that he doesn't have to deal with the recurring bald spots from alopecia. "For me, knowing what *not* to do with the kids I teach—I like to think that's the gift my parents gave me. I can see when a kid is showing signs of anxiety or depression. I see how at this age, some kids who have been struggling to hold it together for so long just can't anymore. Things start to fall apart, and they just can't understand what's happening to them. I *was* that kid."

—

The research on neuroinflammation, pruning, and the brain helps to explain why adverse experiences in childhood are so highly correlated to depression and anxiety disorders in adulthood. It also sheds light on why, according to the National Institute of Mental Health (NIMH), depression affects eighteen million Americans. The World Health Organization recently cited depression as "the leading cause of disability worldwide," responsible for more years of disability than cancer, HIV/AIDS, and cardiovascular and respiratory diseases combined.

This also may explain other brain-based health disorders. For instance, a recent study of brain scans of people suffering from chronic fatigue syndrome, or CFS—myalgic encephalomyelitis, or ME—show higher levels of inflammation in specific parts of the brain, including the hippocampus and amygdala. The greater a patient's level of self-reported CFS symptoms, the greater the degree of visible brain inflammation.

This may also help to account for why it is that those who faced Adverse Childhood Experiences are six times more likely to develop chronic fatigue in the first place.

The Walking Wounded

It's impossible to estimate how many adults who experienced Adverse Childhood Experiences are getting by, day by day, unwittingly navigating a state of low-grade neuroinflammation, functioning despite their "reset tone" in the brain, dealing with general low mood, depression, and anxiety.

This lowered "set point of well-being," this generalized emotional misery, predicts with startling accuracy how likely we are to find ourselves as adults navigating mood fluctuations, anxiety, sadness, fear—reacting to life without resilience, rather than really living life fully.

It's kind of the proverbial cat chasing its tail. Epigenetic changes in life cause inflammatory chemicals to increase. Chronic unpredictable stress sends microglia off kilter. Microglia murder neurons. Neurons die, synapses are less able to connect. Microglia proliferate and create a state of neuroinflammation. Essential gray matter areas of the brain lose volume and tone. White matter—the myelin in the brain that allows for synapses to connect between neurons—is lost. This lack of brain tone impairs thought processes, making negative thoughts, fears, reactivity, and worries more likely over time. An überalert, fearful brain leads to increased negative reactions and thoughts—creating more inflammatory hormones and chemicals that lead to more microglial dysfunction and pruning and chronic inflammation in the brain. The cycle continues.

As McCarthy puts it, "Neuroinflammation becomes a runaway process."

This, she says, "contributes to a chronic overreactivity. Things that most people would get over quickly would send someone with a low level of inflammation into a tailspin. They may not be able to sort out rational thought about what's happening around them—is what's happening right now good, or is it bad? They may be far more prone to see everything as bad."

This is the new psychosocial theory of everything: our early emotional stories determine the body and brain's operating system and how well they will be able to guard our optimal physical and emotional health all of our adult lives.

We take whatever reactive brain and increased sensitivity to stress we develop in childhood with us wherever we go, at any age. We're likely to feel bad mentally and physically a lot of the time. That state of neuroinflammation means we are more likely to walk around in an irritable mood, be easily ticked off and annoyed. Our relationships will suffer. We see hurt where none is intended. We'll likely find the world more aggravating than gratifying. Our chances for a healthy, stable, and satisfying life narrow, and continue to narrow as the years go by. But we can take action to remove the early "fingerprints" that childhood adversity leaves on our neurobiology so that imprint does not stay with us.

The Really Good News

As scientists have learned more about how childhood adversity becomes biologically embedded, they have also learned how we can intervene in this process to reverse the damage of early stress—no matter whether we grew up in a happy, functional family or an often unhappy, dysfunctional one. And no matter what happened to us when we were young.

"The beauty of epigenetics is that it's reversible, and the beauty of the brain is that it's plastic," says McCarthy. "There are many ways that we can immuno-rehabilitate the brain to overcome early negative epigenetic changes so that we can respond normally to both pleasure and pain. The brain can restore itself."

We can heal those early scars to get back to who it is we really are, who we might have been had we not faced so much adversity in the first place. But to do that, we first have to understand why we may be more prone to epigenetic changes than others in the first place, even though we are no less capable of epigenetic reversal and change.

CHAPTER THREE

Why Do Some Suffer
More than Others?

Not everyone's health is sabotaged by unremitting, unpredictable stress in childhood.

Some adults who endured a difficult childhood thrive and are emotionally resilient. For some reason, the past doesn't cast such a long shadow over their lives.

In a Harvard study of elderly people who have enjoyed remarkable longevity, neuropsychologist Margery Silver found that "a particular characteristic that is typical of centenarians" is that they manage life stress very well. Even those centenarians who have "had really very difficult, and even traumatic lives" of extreme adversity—including holocaust survivors—seem to be able to "roll with the punches . . . accept their losses, grieve them and then move on. They bounce back."

Resilient people have what psychologists call "wobble": the ability to waver under the weight of life's suffering and trauma but not fall down. Others fare less well in the face of what life throws their way. The question is: why are some more fragile than others?

Psychiatrists refer to the amount of trauma we experience over the course of our lives, and the cumulative effect of that trauma—how much wear and tear it takes on our body, brain, and mind—as our "allostatic load." The term, coined by Bruce S. McEwen, PhD, professor of neuroendocrinology at Rockefeller University, is derived from "allostasis," the ability to adapt over time to the stressful emotional and physical trials that we encounter, return to a state of equilibrium, and regain our sense of well-being. We wobble, we recover, and we get on with living our lives.

But most kids who experience chronic stress and trauma don't have the tools or maturity to regain their equilibrium. They're just kids caught up in circumstances over which they have little control, trying to make sense of their own confusion and the emotional chaos of the adults around them.

Generally speaking, the higher a child's Adverse Childhood Experiences Score, the higher her allostatic load, and the more likely she will have a high degree of physical and neural inflammation, and that her body and brain may eventually pay a steep physical cost for that early emotional suffering.

When my children were young, we played a game called Elephant, which involves piling planks on top of the elephant's back to build a tower. If you don't place your pieces carefully, the tower starts to sway precariously and topple.

Being a child who endured early, unpredictable stress is a little bit like being that elephant carrying wobbly cargo. Having a lot of early wear and tear can make it harder to bear up under later challenges, and harder to find an interior sense of well-being and solidity—an inner resilience.

Yet some people who've faced a lot of adversity fare better than others. Not every single person with an Adverse Childhood Experience ends up with heart disease, an autoimmune condition, or an anxiety disorder. The correlation is high, but it is not a given.

In his recent book *David and Goliath,* social theorist and researcher Malcolm Gladwell argues that losing a parent in childhood can lead to a mix of both negative and positive outcomes in adulthood, for reasons we don't quite understand. A boy who lost his mom to cancer when he was ten might go on to be a MacArthur genius recipient in cancer research. Such individuals' lives are governed by what Gladwell calls the "Theory of Desirable Difficulty." Struggle strengthens their resolve. It even leads some to do extraordinary and profound things with their lives.

Gladwell researched the personal histories of noteworthy leaders in business, science, and politics and found that in rare cases, there exists an odd benefit of early trauma: "If you take away a mother or father, you cause suffering and despair. But one time in ten, out of that despair arises an indomitable force."

One out of ten is low odds—but that 10 percent is notable. A third of US presidents lost or were distant from a parent. That loss became an impetus for grit and self-reliance, for making something remarkable of themselves. The same applies to a large percentage of British prime ministers and other prominent figures, including Supreme Court justice Sonia Sotomayor, whose alcoholic father died when she was nine.

Of course many leaders who lost or had distant parents in youth also suffered deeply from illness in adulthood, in addition to their great achievements. Abraham Lincoln, who lost his mother in childhood, suffered debilitating bouts of depression. John F. Kennedy, whom biographers cite as having had a cold, preoccupied mother who "never said I love you" or "rumpled his hair," and an overbearing father, suffered from Addison's disease, an autoimmune disease in which the adrenal glands are so overtaxed that they fail to produce the proper steroid hormones. These men were luminous and extraordinary, and we admire them all the more for having led a nation in spite of their private illnesses.

Some might argue that if the pain of having lost a parent or having had a distant, unloving mother or father gives one the extra mental muscles and grit needed to successfully lead a nation, it is a price well paid. But early adversity is far more likely to hold us back. As Gladwell found, nine out of ten people who lose a parent early in life "are crushed by what they have been through." Most kids who have suffered from toxic stress and adverse experiences do not recover without help. And as adults they are all too often still swimming unaware against the hard and invisible current of those emotional forces from long ago, as they try to make their way toward a happy and fulfilling life.

It doesn't matter what type of Adverse Childhood Experience a child faces: all ten categories of ACEs can cause very similar biophysical changes and inflammation. Yet the effect of childhood stress on body, brain, and mind differs for each of us—but not always for the reasons we think it will.

The Theory of Good Wobble

Trauma research shows that the old adage "Whatever doesn't kill you will make you stronger" is rarely true. The more Adverse Childhood Experiences you have, the more likely you are to suffer from later psychological and physical illness. Still, no one waltzes through life without some stress and adversity. And a lack of adversity is not really optimal for healthy development.

At the University at Buffalo, associate professor of psychology Mark D. Seery, PhD, has been searching for the upside of adversity, asking whether some stress exposure might make people stronger over the long term. Seery had hundreds of patients who suffered from chronic, debilitating back pain complete a survey about their lifetime exposure to thirty-seven different types of stressful experiences.

The questionnaire included serious childhood event categories such as a "forced separation from family," or parents' divorce, as well as sexual and physical abuse, all of which echo well-established Adverse Childhood Experiences categories. But he also included a wider range of possible losses and stressors—more ubiquitous stressors such as having experienced the "death of a grandparent," "being discriminated against," or witnessing the "serious illness of a loved one."

Patients who cited a high degree of adversity as children or teens were more likely as adults to frequently visit doctors for chronic back pain. They were also more likely to seek treatment for anxiety or depression.

These findings were in line with other research, but Seery found one surprising difference. "Patients who had experienced absolutely no prior adversity in their childhood fared just as poorly as those who had experienced high levels of adversity," he says. In other words, those participants who had a score of 0 on all childhood adversity questions—including the mild stressors Seery had included—were just as likely to be deeply disabled by their back pain and seek treatment for anxiety or depression as were those who had experienced significant levels of adversity when they were young.

On the other hand, patients who had met up with *some* adversity when they were young, but not too much, were the least likely to be disabled due to back pain later in life, or to later seek treatment for anxiety or depression.

There seemed to be a kind of Goldilocks sweet spot: experiencing just the right dose of hardship as a child or teenager—not too much and not too little—helped build coping skills, resilience, and perspective to meet the challenge of dealing with debilitating, chronic pain later on in one's adult life.

This led Seery to "the idea that experiencing some degree of difficulty can be a good thing, it can prepare us in ways we don't completely understand for later difficulties."

Why did Seery find this upside to adversity in his study, when the same silver lining doesn't appear in Adverse Childhood Experience research? Seery suspects that while "Adverse Childhood Experience research asks respondents about ten big categories of serious traumatic experiences, when we focus on only the most traumatic human experiences, we may miss some folks who have had some trauma, but across a broader array of categories. We miss finding out whether some measure of adversity can actually lead to later resilience."

So Seery tested his hypothesis in another way. He asked respondents to hold their hands in a bucket of very cold water for five minutes. Those who reported a moderate number of negative life events showed less response to physical pain. Seery also had them take a high-stakes test in the lab. And this same group was less likely to have a higher stress response when test taking.

This group also reported less emotional distress and a greater degree of life satisfaction than those who'd experienced a high degree of ACE-like adversity as well as those who'd reported having had no negative life events.

Having faced moderate stress in the past seemed to help individuals cope with newly occurring stressors happening in the here and now, says Seery. "They seemed to have gained a sense that when bad things happen that doesn't mean it's always going to be that bad."

People with no adversity as well as people with a history of high adversity were more likely to be undone by whatever life threw at them, be it chronic back pain, new stressful life events, having their hand submerged in cold water, or taking a high-stakes test. They were the elephants who wobbled while trying to balance the weight they carried, the elephants who were more likely to fall over.

But folks who met up with a moderate number of modestly stressful early adverse life events reported feeling less distress about their lives, showed fewer signs of stress when they encountered new adversity, and had a much higher sense of life satisfaction over time. For these individuals, says Seery, "the adverse events in their past have helped them transition into having more resilience to deal with future events." Their experiences have given them optimal resiliency and well-being. They wobble but they don't fall down.

"Negative life experiences can toughen people, making them better able to manage subsequent difficulties," says Seery. "People who have been through difficult experiences have had a chance to develop an ability to cope."

———

This is not to imply that Adverse Childhood Experiences "do good." They don't. Exposing a child to unpredictable chronic stress causes the body to churn out inflammatory stress hormones igniting a state of chronic physical and neural-inflammation and disease. But moderate stress may be grist for resiliency when it's not deeply personal, chronic, and perpetrated by someone you love.

In other words, watching a grandparent die is stressful, but clearly not your fault. You will likely feel bereft and sad, but are unlikely to interpret it as an event that occurred because you yourself are somehow bad or wrong. The problem isn't about you and who you are.

Recently Jack Shonkoff, MD, director of the Center on the Developing Child and professor at Harvard University, has examined the scientific evidence for the "toxic stress response"—the impact of childhood hardship on brain development and on the development of disease later in life.

"We're at a tipping point in the development of this biological revolution," Shonkoff said at a 2012 forum on toxic stress. "We now understand, in a way we never did before, how early experience literally gets into the body and affects the development of the brain, the cardiovascular system, the immune system, and metabolic systems."

"We're not talking about the need to eliminate stress," he explains. "In children's lives, learning to deal with normative stress is part of healthy development." Normative stress helps kids learn to seek out resourceful strategies, self-soothe, recover, and build the biological capacities for resilience. Toxic stress, however, occurs when a child's stress response systems are activated in the absence of supportive, calming relationships, and stay activated for prolonged periods of time, when that's "basically what life is usually like for a child. This is not the stress associated with a bad day. This is the stress associated with chronic activation of systems that disrupt brain circuits as they're developing, and wear the body down."

Toxic stressors don't toughen up a child—they break down a child's or adolescent's brain so that the child is less able, throughout life, to handle the next thing, and the next. The difference between character-building experiences and toxic stress is really pretty clear.

It's so clear, in fact, that I'll refer to chronic unpredictable toxic stress as childhood CUTS.

A number of factors play into why some children are likely to be more affected by childhood CUTS than others.

The Heavy Price We Pay for Secrets

Most Adverse Childhood Experiences are chronic stressors that happen behind closed doors; parents or other adults may humiliate or tease or mistreat a child in their own living room, or at the dinner table, or in the locker room in ways they wouldn't do at a larger gathering or an event where others are watching. Which means, from a child's perspective, that what is happening is a secret. And as psychologists have long known, when kids feel that something is being kept secret, when no one speaks to them about what's happening or why, but they know that something feels wrong, they assume that it must be bad, and that it must be about *them*. If no one is talking about it, that must mean it's their fault, it must mean that they are the one who *is* bad.

Looking at the sheer numbers, given that 64 percent of kids face a form of severe adversity, there is a good chance that many children are walking around with the vague or pressing sense that something bad is going on, and that they are in some way to blame.

Think of it this way: if you grew up with childhood CUTS, you knew that something wasn't right, even if no one said a word. You likely felt some sense of shame, as if you were, yourself, to blame.

Research bears this out. One recent survey found that nearly 60 percent of adolescents recognized that they were facing, or had faced, at least one category of childhood adversity, even though these teens were only thirteen, fourteen, and fifteen years old. They recognized that they were facing adversity even though they lacked the perspective that they would one day have as adults. And 60 percent of these teens who said they were facing childhood adversity said they'd already faced multiple childhood adversities.

They acknowledged, to researchers, that something that was taking place in their lives was wrong—because researchers asked them the question.

But most kids are never asked. Kat went from the age of five to thirty-five without anyone ever asking her what had happened in her early life. Her past was always "The Big Unmentionable." As a result, she felt "deep-seated shame." Wherever she went, she says, "I carried so much unspoken guilt about what my father had done and about my having said the words that sent my own dad to jail. My family almost never talked about my mom's murder. It was as if none of it had ever happened."

Laura was stuck in a small house with her mother's put-downs. "My mom used to say to me, 'It's you and me against the world,'" Laura says. "It was as if we had this secret together, no matter how crazy it might get, it was just between us. So it never occurred to me, for many years, that in many ways, it was my mom against me."

Kids don't perceive being humiliated or neglected as a moment that holds growth potential. They just know that the family secret they are keeping hurts.

Priscilla, now sixty-one, grew up taking care of her own parents and keeping their secrets. "I grew up surrounded by mental illness," she says. "No one explained it to me. It was never discussed by anyone. I just grew up parenting my parents, as if that were the most normal thing. My dad was a manic-depressive, on lithium, and my mother was a narcissist who needed me to mother her."

When Priscilla was sixteen months old, she had an acute infection. Her fever shot up to 106°F. She began having convulsions in front of her mother. Her parents took her to the hospital, admitted her, and then left her there alone. In the middle of the night, her throat closed up. She was choking for air. A resident walking by her room noticed that Priscilla had stopped breathing and gave her an emergency tracheotomy—without anesthesia. Later, her mother would tell Priscilla the story, over and over, of how scared she had been, rushing her daughter to the hospital, on "the night you almost died," and how her mother felt like *she* might die because she was so scared and unprepared "to have to save my own daughter's life." Priscilla says, "I would have to comfort her about almost losing me. She never thought about how a baby might have felt, having surgery without pain medication, and being left to recover in a hospital alone." That set in place a pattern in which Priscilla handled all of her crises on her own.

"When I broke my collarbone at summer camp when I was eleven, I didn't tell them; it never occurred to me that I *had* parents who could protect me from pain and suffering," she says. "I lived with the pain. When I returned home at the end of the summer, a family friend saw the lump on my chest and told me I had to tell my mother. My mother took me to the doctor. He said it was a case of gross negligence."

But Priscilla didn't resent her parents when she was growing up. "I felt like I was the 'hero child'; I was saving my mom. She was so complimentary, and wanted to be so close to me, I assumed that must be a good thing." It was only as Priscilla came into her teen years that "I began to realize that my mother was living through me; I started to feel emotionally violated by her narcissism. She had to be included in everything I did with my friends, as if she were another teenager. She wanted me to be *her* mother. I began to realize that she didn't love me the way a mother loves a child. She needed me to love *her*, to take care of her since she couldn't get that from her own husband."

Priscilla no longer felt like the hero child. Instead, she says, "I began carrying the weight of this great, shameful secret: really, I had no mother and I never had. I knew, in my heart, there must be something wrong with me. I felt so ashamed that no one *could* love me the way a parent loves a child. I was that unlovable."

When Priscilla turned eighteen, her mother sat her down on the bed and said, "I have been your mother for eighteen years. Now, can you be my mother?" Priscilla recalls "hearing her say those words, but instead of being horrified, I just thought, 'But I have always been your mother . . . why are you asking me this now?'"

During adolescence, Priscilla had begun having panic attacks that were so debilitating, she'd huddle on the floor in the corner of the kitchen or bathroom, sweating, shaking, unable to move or think. "My central nervous system just started collapsing all the time," she says. She was experiencing the kind of "panic disorder that you'd read about soldiers having when they came back from Vietnam, or a woman might have after having been raped. But I hadn't been raped; I didn't go to war. I figured there was just something terribly wrong with me, that this was my fault."

When she went for her college physical, Priscilla was told by a doctor that she had a heart condition, mitral valve prolapse. The valve between her heart's left upper and lower chambers wasn't closing properly. It didn't require treatment, but it would have to be watched, and it was a factor in her panic attacks.

"I had this sense of panic, of wanting something I couldn't have; always wanting it and chasing it, but I'd never get there, I'd never get what I felt I needed to survive."

Priscilla married, had two sons, and in her early fifties became a successful writer, flying around the world to lecture and appear on television. "I perfected the motions of adult living," she says. But beneath it all, "I carried this terrible panic. I had heart palpitations. I felt as if everything could turn into a crisis, which I wouldn't be able to handle, because of my defective nervous system. I felt like a fraud—competent on the outside, but often terrified on the inside. I wasn't living my life at all." Her panic attacks grew worse and more frequent; her husband often had to help comfort her through them.

When Priscilla was well into her fifties, she began to look back at her early family life with more scrutiny. "I started to realize that if I wanted to be who I wanted to be, live the life I wanted to live, I had to stop denying the truth of my childhood. Instead of being at the mercy of my fight-or-flight panic reaction to life, I wanted to learn to surf my central nervous system so that I could learn to surf through life." With meditation and therapy, Priscilla was able to create a calmer frame of mind and markedly decrease her panic attacks as she faced the neglect and vulnerability of her childhood. And she wrote about her search for healing in a redemptive memoir, *Learning to Breathe*.

When children view the adversity they're facing as a "secret" that they need to keep, they're unlikely to reveal what it's like inside their home to an outside adult or to seek help or support beyond the confines of their own dysfunctional family. And without outside support, their Adverse Childhood Experiences will exact a higher physical payment.

The Power of Having Just One Reliable Adult

Children who are more resilient after facing early adversity often had an important, reliable adult to turn to in their youth; a grown-up who stepped in and helped them understand that what was happening wasn't about them and wasn't their fault.

According to Jack Shonkoff's Center on the Developing Child, the presence or absence of adequate adult support, and the duration and nature of a stressor, can make a profound difference in determining whether childhood stressors are tolerable or toxic. Stress is tolerable when longer-lasting difficulties, even serious stressors, such as the loss of a loved one, or a natural disaster, are temporary, limited in duration—and are buffered by relationships with adults who help a child learn to adapt. With someone to lean on, and with love, the brain can recover from what might otherwise be damaging effects.

However, when stressors are strong, frequent, and prolonged—such as chronic neglect, physical or emotional abuse, living with a caregiver who has an addiction or mental illness, or coming of age in a violent environment—and this happens without adequate adult support, stress becomes toxic. Having supportive, responsive relationships with caring adults as early in life as possible makes a profound difference.

Harriet's story illustrates this. Now a forty-eight-year-old lawyer who lives in Austin, Texas, Harriet was raised by a mom who "really didn't know what it meant to parent." When Harriet was four years old, her mother began regularly putting her on an airplane alone to visit her grandfather and her grandmother, both of whom suffered from depression. Harriet's grandfather—her mother's father—"would make me take off my clothes and force me into the bathtub to 'bathe me.'" Harriet still has panic flashbacks to one day, recalling "being naked and afraid, crying, fighting like crazy to get out of that tub; I didn't like what he was doing to me, the way he was bathing me." When she was old enough to later understand what had happened and the implications of it, she told her younger female cousins to stay clear of their grandfather, to never be alone with him. She'd learned to watch out for others, even if no one was watching out for her.

When she was twelve years old, Harriet fell while doing gymnastics; she broke her lower back in two places and didn't tell her mom about the accident, or about how much pain she was in. By the time she was finally seen by a doctor, he asked Harriet, "How are you even walking around?" Because she'd gone untreated, her recovery was never complete, and she was in pain every day of her life.

At the age of sixteen, having recovered from her injury but still living with chronic pain, Harriet was date-raped. Once again, Harriet found herself "naked, fighting, and clawing against a man who wouldn't listen when I asked him to stop." The next day at school, Harriet's "boyfriend" explained the scratches across his face by telling everyone at their high school, "Harriet's a real wildcat in bed!"

Harriet didn't tell her mom what happened then, either. Her mom "would have said, if I'd come to her for help after any of these traumas, 'How could you do this to me, Harriet?' It was always quite clear to me, even at a very young age, that my mother was never going to be a source of comfort to me; I couldn't trust her to help me. If I was afraid, and told her, it quickly became a scene about how I was hurting her with my problems." Indeed, it seems incredible to Harriet now, she says, "that my mom used to put me on that airplane, alone, to go stay with her parents, knowing that they had mental health issues, without ever thinking about what that might mean for me."

When Harriet was nineteen, she told her parents that she thought she was a lesbian, and they disowned her.

By the time Harriet turned thirty, "I was having little tremors all the time," she says. She started to develop a goiter on her neck. She went to see a doctor, who took Harriet's vitals. Harriet's resting heart rate was 140, far higher than it should be. Her doctor ran tests and told Harriet that her thyroid numbers were through the roof—ten times higher than what was considered normal. Harriet had a full-blown case of Graves' disease—an autoimmune disease in which the body's own immune system mistakenly attacks the healthy tissue of the thyroid, causing the thyroid gland to become hyperactive.

At forty-four, Harriet's gynecologist found that she had "a giant, cohesive fibroid located against the posterior side of my uterus, so far back that it was not easily palpated. It had been developing for at least ten years—and it was the size of a baby's head. Only I had no idea, because I was already in so much back pain."

Harriet is not really surprised when I tell her about recent research that shows that girls who are victims of sex abuse are as much as 36 percent more likely to develop uterine fibroid tumors decades later in life.

Looking back, Harriet says, "I see my mother as the context against which everything that was traumatic for me happened." She can't help but wonder how "things might have been different if I'd had a mom to turn to when bad things happened, if I'd felt her support through thick and thin."

—

Clearly, when a child has a reliable parent or adult to turn to, she has a far better chance of being able to make sense of the stress she faces, and, ideally, a smart, stable, caring mentor-adult will intervene on her behalf. Researchers at Emory University recently found that even when children experienced adversity, if they also had a positive family environment, and someone to turn to, they showed changes in an oxytocin receptor gene, which in turn wielded a protective influence, helping those children to be more resilient and better at coping.

—

The good news in Seery's research is that, "Just because something bad has happened to someone, that doesn't mean they're doomed to be damaged from that point on." If we can learn precisely what's giving some individuals who've experienced moderate childhood adversity their resilience, and discern what helps them to interpret their experiences in a way that leads to a greater sense of security and an enhanced ability to cope with life's difficulties, we may be able to apply that understanding more broadly, even years down the road. "It should be possible for people to derive benefits from even higher levels of past adversity, if we know how to help them do so."

When people who have suffered from Adverse Childhood Experiences search out and find healing, they can achieve a beneficial perspective on their lives. And even if we had traumatic experiences, our brains, which, again, are highly malleable and plastic long into adulthood, can build the neural structure for resilience. We can contextualize past trauma in ways that make us even better at dealing with stressful challenges and emerge gracefully in the face of them.

The Sensitivity Gene

Brain development from birth to eighteen is shaped by experiences, but our genetic makeup also influences the way our body and mind perceive and respond to stress. Some people are genetically primed to be more sensitive to what's going on around them in their environment— including any family trauma or hardship they encounter when very young. Others aren't as deeply affected by early adversity; things don't hit them quite so hard. One of the reasons for this difference exists deep within our genetic code.

The Sensitivity Hypothesis explains how and why some people are predisposed to stress reactivity. Roughly 15 percent of the general population possesses a variant of a behavioral gene called 5-HTTLPR, which regulates the neurotransmitter serotonin. Serotonin influences our ability to rebound from emotional trauma and distress. This Sensitivity Gene exists in three variants. People with the short/short variant tend to be highly sensitive to whatever they meet up with in their day-to-day life. When something stressful happens, they may be less able to recover quickly, but they're also more deeply affected by positive influences; when they receive the right kind of nurturance, they do better in life. A mentor who has faith in them or recognizes that they have a gift or skill will profoundly shape them for the better. They soak in the good.

The short/long expression of the serotonin gene doesn't seem to affect people either way very much. However, the long/long expression of this gene is associated with having a greater ability to bounce back from adversity and more easily regain one's footing after stressful events. When bad things happen, those with the long/long variant don't fret or feel it quite so much. What might overwhelm other people in life is the proverbial water off the duck's back. So, they don't end up carrying around such a heavy allostatic load as they go forward in life.

But what's most intriguing about the Sensitivity Hypothesis gene is that it plays a far more profound role in the more vulnerable years of childhood, when the brain is still developing, than it does in how affected we are by stress once we become adults. People with this Sensitivity Gene variant who experience adversity when growing up face the greatest likelihood of suffering from depression in adulthood.

The reason is this: the Sensitivity Gene influences the developing stress response in such a way that, when "sensitive kids" are faced with adversity, their HPA stress axis pumps out even *more* stress hormones. They get a double dose of inflammatory drip from early on, and for a very long time.

In one fascinating study researchers asked several groups of adolescents to perform tasks in a lab setting while receiving ambiguous or negative feedback from observers. One group of teens possessed the short form of the Sensitivity Gene, and had also experienced some type of childhood adversity before the age of six; a second group of teens had the Sensitivity Gene, but hadn't experienced early adversity. Both groups performed tasks such as discriminating between two images on a computer screen that matched or didn't match or playing memory games. They couldn't tell if researchers thought they were doing a good job or not because researchers were intentionally giving them mixed feedback.

The adolescents who carried the Sensitivity Gene and had faced childhood adversity showed more anxiety and made more mistakes while performing the tasks. They assumed that the sometimes discouraging, nonverbal feedback they were getting from evaluators meant they'd done something wrong. These same kids also showed signs of cognitive and emotional difficulties that are associated with later anxiety and depression.

Kids with the Sensitivity Gene who didn't experience childhood adversity didn't show the same reactivity to ambiguous feedback or have trouble regulating emotions. Because they hadn't experienced Adverse Childhood Experiences, the Sensitivity Gene hadn't kicked in.

There are other gene variants that contribute to children's biophysical vulnerability to early stress. Duke researchers found that kids from high-adversity backgrounds who also carried a common gene variant, NR3C1, which, like 5-HTTLPR, makes some children more sensitive to their environment, were much more likely to develop serious problems as adults. This NR3C1 gene, or what we might call the Stress Vulnerability Gene, influences the body's output of cortisol during stress. Seventy-five percent of kids with the stress-reactive variant of this gene developed psychological challenges or addictive behaviors by age twenty-five.

However, when kids with this Stress Vulnerability Gene also received intervention through programs that offered them support, only 18 percent developed psychological disorders and addictions as adults. In other words, the children with the vulnerability gene variant were highly susceptible to stress—but they were also very remarkably responsive to adult help—it made all the difference in their lives.

If you have the Sensitivity Gene or the Stress Vulnerability Gene and faced your share of adverse experiences in childhood, you may find that you are emotionally wired with a hair-trigger stress response. The trajectory of your life may be fraught with more difficulty. For instance, you may be more likely to feel anxiety and fear when a car veers in front of you or someone criticizes your idea at the office or something goes bump in the night. You may have a low-simmering, interior sense that you are not safe. You may pick up on other people's discomfort and anxieties and absorb their stress without even realizing how much it is affecting you and your biology.

Georgia, raised by her cold, controlling mother and a dad with a temper, recalls that she picked up on tension in her home "before arguments even happened," but her sisters were "more oblivious, and a lot tougher." They didn't seem to have the emotional antennae Georgia did. As her sisters neared adolescence, they stood up to her mother and started to "give it right back," Georgia says. "They weren't afraid, sometimes they even went head to head with my mom; they were sassy and exerted their power."

By then, Georgia had already been dubbed by her family as "too sensitive" or "the sensitive one." Labeling her in this way allowed her parents to pretend the tensions in their family were normal, that Georgia was the problem.

"I took in every negative vibe in the family. Eventually, to protect myself, I learned to shut myself down, even if I couldn't shut down my sensors," Georgia says. "By the time I was ten, I'd learned to do what I was told; I made a daily, conscious effort to be as invisible as a human being could possibly be."

When Georgia was thirteen, her mom went to a therapist. Her husband was drinking heavily—and sometimes driving while drunk. Georgia says, "My mother had had a very abusive mother herself, and she'd lost her father whom she'd adored. She was well educated and more or less stuck at home with three small girls. My father told her, 'I'm not paying for therapy, no wife of mine is going to a shrink.'"

Her mom took on a part-time job at a local library to pay for her therapy. She didn't change very much toward Georgia, but, looking back, Georgia appreciates how hard it must have been for her mother to take those steps.

Georgia threw herself into her schoolwork. "I repressed everything except for my intellect." It paid off—her desire to succeed in her own right might even have saved her life. When she was eighteen, Georgia went off to Columbia, where she eventually got her PhD.

Today, at age forty-nine, Georgia wonders a lot "about the multigenerational piece," she says. "My mother's mother was abandoned when she was a baby; my grandmother was very damaged. She was abusive to my mother, who, in turn, was a deeply injured person. The same was true on my father's side—he'd had no real parents who looked out for him. My father's father was depressed and an alcoholic. So was my father." Georgia pauses. "It's as if all those generations of pain landed on *my* back."

"I have a very sensitive system that picks up on what other people can't always sense," she says. "Being able to sense and see what was going on beyond the superficial helped to protect me in a way—I knew when to retreat. But I was also a pain sponge. I absorbed my father's pain, my mother's pain, the pain of their damaged marriage."

As an adult, in addition to degenerative disc disease, depression, and fibromyalgia, Georgia has also faced trouble in her relationships. She married in her early twenties, hoping to rewrite her own family's unhappy story by creating a more loving and supportive home of her own—a safe haven.

But the marriage didn't last. Georgia found it difficult to communicate and voice her feelings and needs honestly, as did her husband. Over time, lack of communication broke down their relationship. After she divorced, Georgia came to have this "strong inner vision" that there had to be a very different way of loving and living than what my parents had demonstrated for me. If I couldn't find that road, I didn't know if life was really worth it. I knew I either had to get on a journey toward physical and emotional healing or fold it all up and pack it in."

Despite everything Georgia knows about her childhood, she finds it "daunting" to answer yes to several ACE questions but relieved to know that she "wasn't 'too sensitive' all those years," after all.

Georgia's descriptions of her childhood illustrate the Sensitivity Hypothesis and the Vulnerability Hypothesis at work: some children see more, perceive more, know more, feel more. These are the same children who may carry even deeper psychic wounds from their adversity-laden childhood, and who may grow up to face more pressing physical and emotional symptoms in the future. This doesn't mean that what happened was less traumatic than they think it was; it means that they felt the pain of it more deeply.

Still, the Sensitivity Gene brings with it distinct neurobiological pluses. The same plasticity of the brain that makes sensitive children highly reactive to stress also makes them more intuitive and receptive, more easily shaped by what is good and healthy in their environment, too: the support they're shown, the loving relationships they experience, the caring mentor who sees something special in them and takes them under his or her wing. Even later efforts in adulthood to reshape and rehabilitate their own brains may bring them greater healing results.

When "sensitive" children experience a supportive, nurturing childhood, they actually show the *fewest* signs of depression in later life, even compared to those with the long/long version of the gene. They become even more likely than other people to develop positive and beneficial psychological characteristics, and to thrive. Even after suffering as children, their adult behaviors are still malleable, which translates into a profound ability to change after they become adults, despite their history. Regardless of what happened when you were young, regardless of your sensitivity, if you set out to rehabilitate your brain and downshift your stress reactivity, you have a very good chance of doing so.

Georgia is sensitive; her intuitive makeup made her childhood more painful; but that same inner, creative sensitivity is what gave Georgia her "strong inner vision" that life *could* be different. And that inner vision would later propel Georgia on a transformative healing journey as an adult.

The Sensitivity Gene can make you more adept at learning how to deal with life's inevitable suffering, and help you to learn to turn the fallout of childhood adversity into grist for remarkable self-growth.

The Perception Puzzle

Kelly McGonigal, PhD, a Stanford University psychologist, has revealed a fascinating relationship between the perception of stress, illness, and resilience, through her work on a study that followed thirty thousand adults for eight years. The study asked two questions: "How much stress have you experienced in the last year?" and "Do you believe that stress is harmful for your health?"

Not surprisingly, those who had experienced a lot of stress in the past year had a much higher rate—a 43 percent risk—of dying. More stress means more inflammation, more illness, and death. But, says McGonigal, "the relationship between stress and early death was only true for people who *also* believed that stress is harmful to your health. People who experienced a lot of stress but who did not view stress as harmful were no more likely to die." In fact, she points out, this latter group "had the lowest risk of dying of anyone in the study, including people who had relatively little stress."

Research on "perceived stress" tells us it isn't a stressful experience that causes you harm; it's your reaction to that feeling of stress that's most harmful.

When we are able to reframe stress in our minds, and recognize that feeling anxious can actually be a useful reaction, we lessen the harmful long-term effects of stress itself. When you understand that your "pounding heart is preparing you for action," says McGonigal, and the fact that you're breathing harder is a sign that oxygen is pumping into the brain in order to help you think faster, you realize that the "stress response is helpful for your performance; it's helping you to rise to a challenge." With that recognition, your stress response becomes far less physiologically damaging to your body. Tightened blood and heart vessels relax, the body relaxes—and yet you retain the benefits of the stress response: a heightened awareness.

When we believe a stress response is aiding us, by alerting us to the fact that we need to take action or get help, we are also more likely to seek out support and take steps to surround ourselves with and open up to people who care about us. When we act on that instinct to seek social contact and support, we generate more oxytocin—the compassion hormone. Oxytocin protects our bodies from the effects of stress even more. Oxytocin, McGonigal points out, "is a natural anti-inflammatory."

Children, of course, are too vulnerable and young to reframe how they view adversity, especially if the person causing their trauma is a caregiver. But adults can take some heart from McGonigal's research into perceived stress. If you can perceive past stressors in your childhood as catalysts to your growing into who you hope to become, that reframing can be a critical step in your personal journey in healing, forgiveness, and transformation.

In reframing the past, it can help to remember that while what happened when you were young was no doubt wrong, even unbearable, more often than not, that pattern of family dysfunction was set in place long before you were born; the adversity you suffered was the indirect result of the childhood Chronic Unpredictable Toxic Stress that your own parents endured, and their parents faced.

As Harriet acknowledges, her mother grew up amid her own toxic multigenerational legacy of Adverse Childhood Experiences. "Looking back, I realize my mom never had a chance of being a calm and loving mother, given her own history," Harriet says. "I don't blame her. She didn't have the tools."

Rashomon Revisited—or How We Remember

The way in which we store our memories in the brain—and replay them over time—is another important factor in how we are affected by childhood adversity.

Four siblings in a family can have four entirely different ideas about what happened twenty years ago when Mom and Dad divorced, taking different sides on the issue, rehashing their reasons for feeling the way they do. As in the movie *Rashomon*, each sees the events of the past differently, drawing different conclusions.

Georgia says that when she and her sisters discuss their childhood, they can't agree on what growing up was really like. Georgia feels her sisters don't validate her experiences; they feel that Georgia overemphasizes the negative aspects of life when they were kids, is still overreacting, and can't let go of the past.

Some of this difference in how we remember is genetic; part of it is due to the fact that each child in a family has different experiences within family life, and some is also due to how the brain stores longterm memories and reshapes them over time.

The brain's ability to remember a fear or trauma response has been crucial to the survival of our species. As our ancestors evolved, they had to be able to remember, for instance, that certain berries are toxic and make them sick. So they made a lifelong association between the berry and severe illness. Every time they saw that red berry, they thought, don't eat it, you could die.

When we have suffered Chronic Unpredictable Toxic Stress, simply remembering a person or event that was hurtful or humiliating may trigger us to relive that earlier hurt in vibrant detail—and cause us to experience a similar deep-fear response again. We don't want to be reexperiencing that stress, and yet all too often our worst memories are those we recall the most.

Why are these memories so potent, even when we don't want them to be?

Specific hormones dramatically change developing brain synapses when we feel fear, love, or rage. When something traumatic occurs, the hormone noradrenaline—the brain's equivalent of adrenaline—alters the chemical and electrical pathways in the areas of the brain responsible for memory formation. These hormones trigger a complex biochemical process in which the brain captures, stores, and encodes these traumatic memories—a process neuroscientists refer to as "consolidation." That's why our most robust human memories—our vivid autobiographical snapshots from childhood—are associated with strong emotional events during which we felt potent fear, anxiety, love, humiliation, or rage.

Most people consider powerful memories to be like snapshots or video clips that we can review and replay, and assume our memories are a true rendition of the past.

But those captured memories actually get revised all our lives. Even after a memory has been consolidated—encoded and stored in our amygdala and hippocampus—it doesn't *stay* consolidated. Our brain rewrites those memories over time, based on new information and experiences. Each time we remember an incident of childhood adversity, that particular memory becomes labile, or susceptible to changes in how and what we remember about what happened.

Neuroscientists call this process "memory reconsolidation" because we continually update and revise our existing memories as time goes by. We rewrite some details based on new input, erasing others.

And yet, that memory is always encapsulated by the same feelings we felt when the experience first occurred, at whatever age we were at the time. For instance, each time Harriet recalls how her grandfather forced her into the bathtub, she reexperiences that five-year-old's feeling of vulnerability, that same terrible sense of rage, helplessness, and shame she felt then. When we mentally revisit an event, we are always that young age.

Without realizing it, we make a lot of our life decisions based on powerful, key life memories. Big events become family stories of moral import passed down from generation to generation, affecting family dynamics. Families can even break down and break apart over differing ideas of what happened decades ago, and who was to blame. We learn not to be taken advantage of in business because of what Uncle so-and-so did to our mom. We avoid certain types of people and situations because of the time our dad had that incident in his youth that he tells us changed the trajectory of his life.

But to some degree, memory plays hoaxes on us all. The thing you are so very certain about—the black stiletto heels your mother was wearing on the fateful day she told you she was leaving your father— may not have been black stilettos after all. You simply added that detail years later, based on later input; on another occasion when she was angry with you and yelling, she was wearing black heels. You've rewritten your earlier memory to add in "stiletto heels." You've layered more onto the original memory.

Our brains construct a world that no one else can see, touch, or hear. Or, as Buddhist teachers sometimes say, "The truth is a pathless land."

This is not to say that your memories are wrong, or that you are wrong to put great store in them. But you are not the same person you were yesterday, because what happened yesterday changes you. And it even changes how you perceive what happened forty years ago.

We store memories in two ways: in explicit or implicit memory.

"Explicit memory" is the recollection of specific events, details, concepts, and ideas. The greater the sense of danger or pain, the more neurons fire and wire together, registering an experience in an explicit memory.

An "implicit memory" is the emotional sense of how events have made us feel; it's our gut response when we think about something. Many kids who've faced childhood adversity carry forward implicit memories from the first few years of life—when they were too young to even remember the explicit details of what happened. Harriet, for instance, recently found hospital records that showed that she was hospitalized for "dehydration" during her first two years of life—multiple times. She doesn't remember those hospitalizations, or feeling thirsty, or weak and dehydrated, but finding these documents helped her to understand why she had such a visceral sense that her mother never protected her or kept her safe. The implicit memory that she was in danger is there, along with all the explicit memories that she recalls from growing up with her mom.

Indeed, in understanding childhood adversity, the accuracy of who was wearing what or where people were standing is far less important than the fact that something emotionally or physically harmful happened that caused the inflammatory stress response to kick in.

Kat was five when she saw her mother on her father's office floor, and has recalled that scene thousands of times in her life. She knew what happened. Even if over the years she started to reimagine her mom's shoes in a different color, she still knew what had happened. The scene was not less true. She felt, deep within, the bigger picture of what was taking place.

Early memories of raw, emotional intensity cause neurons to wire and fire together, and they get tweaked continually over time. These memories have a potent draw on us all our lives, and we revisit and think about that thing that happened when we are eleven throughout our lives—when we are thirty, or forty, or even sixty-five.

As the Buddhist teacher Thich Nhat Hanh says, "There is a tendency to want to go back to the past. Regret and sorrow are always there to draw us back."

———

Yet, instead of getting caught in replaying mental videos of what happened in the past, we need to work it through so that we don't imbue that past adversity with more emotional content over time. Working through these memories is important because strong memories condition us to be on alert for similar situations in the future—which means we're always on alert, watching for the next adverse situation in which we might be made to feel the same way we felt as children. We're consciously and unconsciously looking for more information in order to reconsolidate that memory, continually updating our understanding of how and when and why such situations represent danger.

That can be a real problem, because the brain's alert center, the amygdala, operates much faster than the brain's cortex. It takes two hundred milliseconds for the amygdala to compute, based on our past memories, whether to trigger fight or flight, compared with three to five seconds for the cortex to make a more judicious decision and weigh what's happening—which means our memories can influence us to have a knee-jerk reaction before we think. If your boss is wearing the same perfume that your narcissistic, borderline mother wore, or if she wears black high heels that click in the same way as your mom's did on the parquet floor, or if she's a bit hypercritical in a way that reminds you of your mother's passive-aggressive jabs, your brain is going to sense danger, register fight or flight, and you're going to have trouble reacting to your boss as your boss.

Our brain is hyperbusy looking for confirmation that the world is a scary and dangerous place, and so are the people in it. We begin to overgeneralize our fearful memories, which can lead to generalized anxiety, worsening our set point of well-being.

When you are drawn back again and again into the past without taking steps toward healing, recovering from childhood wounds can prove difficult, if not impossible. Exploring your adverse experiences, telling your story, in order to understand and better work through the past, is a crucial step in healing.

The good news is that, as we will see in Chapter Seven, researchers have been using this new understanding of the constantly evolving process of reconsolidating our past memories to understand how we might revisit painful memories in ways that finally remove their power over us. We can become more like those centenarians that Harvard researchers studied, who wavered under the weight of life's suffering, grieved for their losses, and then moved on with their lives.

Meanwhile, as we will see in the next chapter, among the many factors that affect how Adverse Childhood Experiences will influence your body and brain, perhaps the most important one of all is the sex that you were born.

CHAPTER FOUR

The Female Brain on Adversity: The Link to Autoimmune Disease, Depression, and Anxiety

Kendall is fifty-two, a wife, mom, and marketing consultant with an Ivy League degree who describes herself as having been a "small, underweight child in a family full of beautiful people." When her parents were dating, they were known as the "Ken and Barbie" of their state university, where her dad played baseball. Kendall's dad became a patent attorney, her mom worked as a professional model. Kendall's older brother and younger sister were star athletes, part of the beautiful-people club.

Appearances really were pretty much "everything," and her family didn't quite know what to do with Kendall. She was told by her mother that she'd been ill with severe colic as a baby and was always crying. "Comforting me didn't work, so they let me just cry it out." Kendall was so tiny that she and her sister, who was two years younger, were taken to be twins.

Because she was different, Kendall was teased and subjected to a kind of under-the-radar hazing that was "sanctioned by my whole family."

Strikingly pretty today, Kendall resembles a dark-haired Meryl Streep with broad cheekbones; large, inviting green eyes; and brown hair that she pulls into a ponytail. Growing up, she was often told that despite being "sickly," she "had a cute face." And that one small thing, she says, "probably saved me."

By the time Kendall was in grade school, she routinely had terrible stomach cramps and nausea, and often felt so fatigued and weak that it was hard to go to school. "The overarching memory of my childhood is my parents telling me to 'stop whining and complaining.'" she says. In a photo album from Kendall's childhood, there are pictures of her with her family; her brother, sister, and parents stand with their arms at their sides—while Kendall clutches what looks to be her bloated stomach, covering it tightly with both hands.

By the time she was ten, Kendall was having chronic diarrhea. Her skin was pale, anemic. That year, her mom was in the midst of planning a big family vacation. "I told my mom that something wasn't right, that my throat hurt, my stomach hurt, and I was so tired all the time. But she said, 'Stop this nonsense! Stop trying to be the center of my attention!'"

It was a very long time, Kendall says, before "my mother got around to taking me to the doctor." When the doctor saw Kendall, he told her mother that Kendall had strep and tonsillitis and very low blood pressure. Blood tests revealed that she had acute anemia, which required immediate treatment.

Her family went on their planned vacation skiing in Canada and took Kendall along. She was on antibiotics and iron pills. "My parents expected me to carry my skis on my back, and trudge back up the mountain. In our family, if you were sick, people acted as if you'd done something wrong. You were weak; you needed to buck up.

"I remember walking up the mountain and feeling as if I were going to fall facedown in the snow, just willing my legs to get me to the lift."

She recalls finding her way back to their room, "where I just lay on top of my bed shivering and shivering. No one came." Finally, she says, "my mother came in our room and yelled, 'Don't you even know how to take care of yourself!' "

After Kendall ran out of iron pills, her mother assumed her daughter must be fine, and didn't follow up with the doctor. That year Kendall began to show signs of obsessive-compulsive disorder. Sometimes, she says, "I would spin around in circles to just calm myself down. One day, I told my mom, 'I can't stop spinning, I want to stop but I *can't*,' and my mom stared at me, then turned around and walked out of the room."

One night, Kendall recalls, "right before we sat down at the dinner table, my dad started spinning in front of my brother and sister as if to mimic me, and my brother and sister doubled over, laughing. I had to sit there and pretend that nothing was happening, or they would have made fun of me for getting upset."

There was never a sense that the way she was being marginalized was wrong, or that she needed help for her chronic stomach problems or anxiety. Instead, "they had all decided I was crazy and it was okay to make fun of me; I was fair game, the weak runt in the bunch."

Once, Kendall reported to the school nurse, who called Kendall's mother to tell her that Kendall had a high fever and had to be picked up. She heard her mom's voice, through the nurse's phone, say sharply, "Well, she better really be sick!" When her mom came to get her, she said, "You couldn't just manage to get through school for two more hours, I had to come and get you in the middle of the day?"

Her parents were victims of generations of their own dysfunctional family dynamics. "My father's mother committed suicide when he was a boy, and his family never talked about it. It was not to be discussed." Kendall says this explains "why my father worshipped my mother, and never questioned how unloving she was. I think he needed to worship her as a mother figure, because he was still searching for the perfect mom, the mom who wouldn't leave *him*. So he always took my mom's side rather than tarnish his ideal image that she was such a great mother, the mother he never had." In fact, her dad's frequent refrain was, "Mothers are the center of this universe, and don't you forget it."

"I wasn't fitting in with their perfect picture; I was ruining it, and it made them so mad," Kendall says.

As Kendall became a teen, her health problems worsened. Nausea and diarrhea became constant.

She was twelve when her sister and brother made up a nickname for her: "Kits." It was an acronym for "Kendall Is a Toilet Sitter," words they would chant because she was so often in the bathroom. Her siblings took to calling her "Kits" all the time. Her parents never said a word. Meanwhile, "my parents had a different nickname for me: 'Camille.' They'd taken the name from the Greta Garbo movie in which the main character spends the entire film dramatically coughing while dying of tuberculosis. If I said I was tired, my parents would sigh and say, 'Oh, there goes our Camille.' Or, they might just say outright, 'stop faking, stop whining, stop being a drama queen, stop milking this.'"

Around that time, a college baseball player who her dad had been mentoring moved in with Kendall's family. He was from a troubled background, but was a star player, who needed a home, her mother told them. One day, the young man was visibly upset, and, Kendall says, "I'll never forget watching my mom sit down and gently and kindly calm him down and soothe him. It was painful to watch my mom shower this boy we barely knew with the kind of love and affection and warmth she'd never shown me. Keeping the superstar athlete happy and healthy for the sake of the team was more important than whether her own daughter was thriving or not."

Despite all this, Kendall says, "I went into my twenties thinking that my parents had been fine. They were beautiful; we'd lived a life of luxury and travel. They took care of my college. I didn't think about whether what I'd experienced was normal; I assumed I'd had a great childhood and *I'd* been a problem kid. I felt so much shame about who

I was, about my secret bathroom problems and anxiety. As soon as I entered a building or got on a plane, I'd zero in on where the bathroom was. I wasn't normal.

"I had internalized my mother's vision of me; that the thing that was wrong wasn't a health-related problem—what was wrong was *me*. My terrible weakness of character."

It would be years before Kendall would wonder, "Why did my mother never try to solve my health problems, why did she never once say, 'Wow, what's going on here, how can I help my child?' "

When she was twenty-two, and had just graduated from university, Kendall took a job in a social worker's office as a receptionist. "One day I saw a girl about twelve or thirteen years old come into the office with a mom who looked worried and the girl was spinning and spinning. I asked someone in the office, 'Is that something people get treated for?' And they said, 'Yes, that's a sign of obsessive-compulsive disorder.' "

That revelatory moment stayed with her. Kendall took a job as a corporate event planner and by the time she was in her midtwenties, she was ushering groups of international business travelers around the world, "going to great lengths to hide my diarrhea and nausea, my OCD and massive panic attacks. Underneath everything I did I was so afraid that if I was sick, no one would love me, so I hid any aspect of myself that didn't appear perfectly healthy and well." Kendall had "a primal fear of being tainted, unlovable, and imperfect."

There was one highlight in her life, "an older woman, a former neighbor who had actually known my parents and my family when I was growing up, who had moved to the same city I was living in, not far from me. We would sometimes meet for coffee." This older woman had "done a lot of work in therapy. She had witnessed, up close, what my life was like growing up. She knew certain details about my family, the fact that my grandmother had killed herself, my father's drinking."

One day this older woman confessed to Kendall "that when my siblings and I were little kids, my father had had a 'fairly serious depressive episode,' and she had worried about my father's 'scary rages.'" Learning that someone who knew her family didn't see her parents as perfect, but flawed, was "completely eye-opening."

Still, Kendall had been so brainwashed by her upbringing that she didn't take herself to the doctor even after she became an adult. She married at thirty-five, and after the birth of her first child, she hit a new physical low. "I was dizzy and weak. I could basically only get around for a few hours a day. The rest of the time I had to lie down. There was very little food I could keep down. And I worried, How am I going to take care of my baby?"

At one point, she was driving with her baby daughter in the car when she began vomiting. She had to pull over.

Kendall was terrified. "I had been brought up to believe that there was not an option for me to be sick. Mothers of young children often feel they are not allowed to be sick, but my conditioning went way beyond that. I felt that I had to get better immediately, or I didn't deserve to exist. I needed to find a way to get functional fast because I was otherwise disgraceful and unfit. If I was sick and couldn't be well, the only alternative was annihilation."

Finally, Kendall got to the point that she was vomiting almost every day, and she saw a doctor.

He was shocked at her condition. It didn't take her doctor long to tell Kendall that he suspected she had a "textbook case of celiac disease."

Her tests came back positive for celiac, an autoimmune disease in which the body develops autoantibodies against the gluten in food that enters the gut, and those autoantibodies attack not just the gluten but destroy the lining of the gut itself. She was also severely anemic.

After taking her patient history, her doctor asked her, "How is it that no one has ever helped you?"

Kendall was also making autoantibodies against her own thyroid—she had autoimmune thyroiditis. Her doctor diagnosed her with vasovagal syncope, a disorder of the autonomic nervous system that can lead to fainting and seizing and profound fatigue. Overnight, Kendall went from a lifetime of being told she was a Camille and a "toilet sitter" to having four diagnoses: two autoimmune diseases, vasovagal syncope, and anemia.

Her doctor put her on outpatient iron infusions at the local hospital. Then she was diagnosed with a third autoimmune disease: Sjögren's syndrome, a rheumatological autoimmune condition.

At first, Kendall rationalized that celiac disease might not have been easily diagnosed twenty-five years earlier, when she'd been very young. But, according to her doctor, her case was unusually clear-cut; even a pediatric gastroenterologist "back then" might well have picked up on it, if Kendall's parents had sought medical care for her. At the very least, if she'd been taken to a specialist, she would have been diagnosed with an inflammatory bowel disorder, encouraged to make dietary changes, and given regular iron supplements.

Today, Kendall explains, "What I experienced all those years ago was gross medical neglect by my own parents. It's still hard to get my hands around the fact that what was happening was wrong. It is very elusive to hold on to the fact that this was not all somehow my fault."

———

Kendall and I first corresponded after she read a piece I had written about the relationship between childhood adversity and adult illness. When I first talked to Kendall after receiving her emails, she told me, "The first time I read what you wrote about the link between what happened in childhood and being ill as an adult, I just felt stunned. I kept rereading the words. It was one of the most eye-opening moments of my life. I knew inside, *This is true for me*. I knew it in the core of my being.

"I realized that what had happened to me had done a lot of emotional damage, but I didn't get that it had also done *physical* damage," she explains. "I've always thought that if you hadn't experienced sexual or physical abuse, then you had nothing to complain about. But as far as your immune system is concerned, it doesn't matter what the source of your stressor is. Your immune system can't tell the difference. And, really, as a kid, neither could I."

Kendall recognizes that she might also have had a genetic proclivity to both celiac and OCD—"but the humiliations and neglect I'd experienced my whole childhood turned what might have been a lit match into a raging fire."

Kendall has an Adverse Childhood Experiences Score of 6.

"I am trying not to be angry or blame my parents," she says. "I was a small, sensitive child who took the brunt of generations of neglect, the same maltreatment and lack of nurturing that my parents endured themselves when they were young. And they passed all that along to me—because that is exactly what they had been trained to do."

Many women with a history of childhood adversity develop a constellation of anxiety and depressive disorders, and autoimmune disease, and they do so in far greater numbers than men. This is certainly worrisome in and of itself. But it's made more so by another factor: women experience more adversity in childhood in the first place.

When Vincent Felitti, MD, and Robert Anda, MD, first published their Adverse Childhood Experiences study findings, Felitti was shocked to discover that women were "50 percent more likely than men to have experienced five or more categories of Adverse Childhood Experiences."

And the more ACEs one has, the greater the likelihood of later neural and physical inflammation and disease.

Felitti believes that "toxic childhood stress lies behind mainstream medicine's attitude that women are naturally prone to ill-defined health problems such as fibromyalgia, chronic fatigue syndrome, obesity, irritable bowel syndrome, and chronic pain." Other disorders, including more than one hundred autoimmune diseases, also blindside and sideline women in the prime of their lives far more than they afflict men. Heads of clinics at major hospitals and top researchers often say that American women in midlife suffer from chronic health disorders—autoimmune disease, depression, migraines, chronic fatigue, fibromyalgia, bowel disorders, back pain—in such greater numbers than men that American women in midlife might well be called "the walking wounded of our day." Yet the link between childhood pain and adult female ill health remains unrecognized in medical circles, contributing to what Felitti says is an ongoing "medical blindness" to the social realities of the impact of a woman's gender on her health and lifelong well-being.

Research on Adverse Childhood Experiences provides an understanding as to why this relationship between early adversity and chronic immune mediated diseases in women is so strong. In childhood, the female body and brain react and change in response to stressors in ways that are different from the male brain and body's reactions.

Girls, Early Adversity, and the Autoimmune Connection

To find out more about the correlation between childhood Chronic Unpredictable Toxic Stress and autoimmune disease in women, I turned to DeLisa Fairweather, PhD, associate professor of toxicology at the Johns Hopkins Bloomberg School of Public Health and Mayo Clinic, one of today's reigning experts on women, sex differences, and autoimmune disorders. Fairweather is coauthor, with Vincent Felitti and Robert Anda, of a landmark study that examined 15,357 adults who had enrolled in the original Kaiser/CDC study on Adverse Childhood Experiences in 1995. Fairweather looked at each ACE Study participant's medical records to see if there was a relationship between having had Adverse Childhood Experiences and later being diagnosed and hospitalized with an autoimmune disease.

Fairweather and I meet at a downtown Baltimore restaurant to talk about her findings. She is short, brunette, and so affable a lunch date, you'd hesitate to peg her as a lab director who spends eleven-hour days managing a toxicology lab and writing grants. She has an infectious enthusiasm for science.

In her study of Adverse Childhood Experiences, Fairweather looked at just twenty-one of the most common autoimmune conditions, including rheumatoid arthritis, lupus, and thyroiditis. The initial results were shocking. "The relationship between ACEs and autoimmune disease, particularly in women, was so striking that we feared no one would believe our numbers." She says, even after the data were checked and double-checked, "We found that a remarkable, disproportionate number of individuals who had experienced childhood adversity were later hospitalized for an autoimmune condition—and a disproportionate number of these individuals were women. The more childhood adversity a woman had, the higher her risk became, and the more likely she was to end up in the hospital at some point in her adult life in order to be treated for an autoimmune condition."

For every ACE Score a woman had, her likelihood of being hospitalized with any one of these twenty-one autoimmune diseases increased by 20 percent. For instance, a woman with three Adverse Childhood Experiences had a 60 percent greater chance of being hospitalized with an autoimmune disease than a woman with none.

For every ACE Score a man had, his chances of being hospitalized for an autoimmune disease increased 10 percent—also a very significant and disturbing correlation. Still, the risk that childhood adversity would lead to an autoimmune disease that was so serious it required hospitalization in adulthood was twice as high for women as it was for men.

"Stress causes autoimmune symptoms to become worse," says Fairweather. "So if any chronic inflammatory disease could be linked to early childhood stress, we figured it would be autoimmune diseases. But we were completely unprepared for how powerful the relationship would turn out to be."

In many other studies, Fairweather continues, "in order to see the relationship between ACEs and chronic disease, you might have to look at patients who had four or five ACEs to see such a significant correlation. But with autoimmune diseases, we saw a very notable increase even among women who had had only two ACEs."

Fairweather confesses that the link she found was so stark that she and her colleagues decided not to report the relationship between women who had more than two Adverse Childhood Experiences and their likelihood of developing autoimmune disease. "The correlation was so significant for those with higher ACE Scores that we didn't think anyone would *believe* us—you just don't see such extreme relationships reported in the scientific literature."

Take Kendall, with her ACE Score of 6. According to Fairweather, Felitti, and Anda's research, Kendall's chance of having an autoimmune disease once she reached adulthood was 140 percent greater than that of a woman who had experienced no Adverse Childhood Experiences at all. And, in fact, Kendall at fifty-two was diagnosed with three autoimmune diseases.

Indeed, if you are diagnosed with one autoimmune disease, you are at a three-times-greater risk of developing other autoimmune diseases.

This link between being female, facing adversity in childhood, and later developing a serious autoimmune disease is so consequential that it resembles the link between smoking and lung cancer, drunk driving and car accidents, and unprotected sex and pregnancy.

Fairweather and her colleagues also found that one in three adults who had faced adversity prior to the age of eighteen was admitted into the hospital for an autoimmune condition some thirty years later— and this was especially true for rheumatic autoimmune diseases such as lupus, rheumatoid arthritis, and Sjögren's syndrome. And, says Fairweather, "80 percent of these patients were women."

Other studies from around the world also bear out this striking relationship between childhood adversity and autoimmune disease in adulthood. While autoimmune diseases strike women three times more than men, for certain illnesses, that ratio is even higher. Women suffer from Hashimoto's thyroiditis at a rate of 10:1 compared with men. In lupus, that rate is 9:1. In Sjögren's syndrome, 9:1. In antiphospholipid syndrome, 9:1. In primary biliary cirrhosis, 9:1. Autoimmune disease is one of the top ten leading causes of death in women under the age of sixty-five.

Although Fairweather, Felitti, and Anda did not include multiple sclerosis in their study sample, researchers recently found that patients with MS score significantly higher on the Childhood Trauma Questionnaire. The association between experiencing early life stress and later developing MS—another autoimmune disease that primarily strikes women—is compelling.

To best understand Fairweather's findings, we need to remember the basic physiological differences between women and men. Women are, generally, physically smaller than men and our hearts and lungs are much smaller in size. Yet our anatomy makes added room to carry a fetus in order to create new human life.

"Our smaller heart, lungs, and other organs still have to be able to do everything a human male does—pump oxygen, circulate blood, run fast, think fast, be awake sixteen or seventeen hours a day—and have the necessary fuel to carry a child to term so that it can survive outside the womb," says Fairweather. Do double duty, on half the machinery.

Women can do so much more on so much less partly because we have much higher baseline levels of the hormone estrogen than men do. Estrogen, which is really a catchall phrase for several hormones, acts as a kind of chemical messenger, carrying information and instructions from one group of our cells to another. It's produced not only in female ovaries but also in our adrenal glands.

Women also have higher baseline levels of glucocorticoids, or GCs—which include the steroid-hormone cortisol. GCs, including cortisol, help to protect women by increasing our ability to regulate inflammation—at least when our fight-or-flight stress response is functioning properly.

For instance, if we have a sudden injury, or have to fight off an infection, glucocorticoids help to reduce that inflammation by suppressing proteins that would promote more inflammation. Extra help from GCs in regulating inflammation ensures that pregnant women who have to deal with sudden inflammation won't miscarry; it's nature's way of making sure that we keep our embryo safe and carry it until term, even if we are hurt or ill. Our immune system is poised, all the time, to protect our ability to carry another life.

This is the upside to having a more pronounced and robust cortisol response than men, at least when our stress reactivity is working well. Estrogen also helps the immune system produce fighter antibodies. Antibodies go after any foreign invader, such as a virus or bacteria.

This is why, says Fairweather, "when women have the flu, or get a vaccine, we have a different, more robust immune response to infection and immunization than men do; we develop a greater antibody response."

On the downside, estrogen can also increase the number of autoantibodies women have. And autoantibodies—antibodies that turn against you and attack the body itself—attack and tear down organs and tissue in every known autoimmune disease.

Multiple, chronic stressful events lead to changes in the developing brain that dysregulate our inflammatory response, allowing inflammation to flourish and build, slowly and silently. The fact that women have a higher baseline level of glucocorticoids complicates things, says Fairweather. "Men start with lower baseline levels of cortisol, so when stressful events happen, cortisol levels have to rise faster in order to help men to successfully regulate inflammation."

In contrast, women already have higher baseline levels of glucocorticoids, because of estrogen. "Normally, when women are healthy and unstressed, we have a more protective cortisol response," says Fairweather. But when women—and especially girls—face stressful events and the inflammatory response becomes dysregulated, something happens in us that doesn't happen in men: Our high levels of GCs go down. Our bodies become a lot *less* able to regulate inflammation.

As girls begin to come into puberty, at around age ten, they also start to have higher levels of estrogen, so they start to produce higher levels of antibodies and autoantibodies. This equation means that when women face chronic ongoing stress, our glucocorticoids stop properly regulating inflammation. At the same juncture, our estrogen is still high, which means autoantibodies can run amok.

High autoantibodies, low system controls. This combination, says Fairweather, "vastly increases the likelihood that girls will grow up to later develop an autoimmune disease, especially a rheumatic autoimmune disease like lupus or Sjögren's syndrome."

You might think of it this way: GCs are like the castle gate that's lowered over a moat to keep those in the castle safe, to allow in just the right number of soldiers, or antibodies, and to keep out rogue mercenaries—or autoantibodies. Girls make more of these rogue autoantibodies, which are elevated by estrogen. But when girls face chronic ongoing early stress, normally protective GCs aren't able to do the job. The castle gate starts to give way, allowing, in this case, damaging rogue autoantibodies to begin an all-out attack.

Fairweather adds, "It takes time for inflammation and autoantibodies to cause damage to organs in the weeks, months, and years after a stressful event. A child can undergo chronic stress at twelve, and it can take thirty years or longer for the immune damage caused by that chronic adversity to progress to a clinically recognizable disease."

At that late date, the correlation between that stressed little girl and the ill woman is obvious to neither the patient nor her physician.

The fact that women have more estrogen as they enter the teen years may not be the only explanation. According to Margaret McCarthy, PhD, professor of neuroscience at the University of Maryland School of Medicine, male resilience may stem from the male immune response, which "is programmed by high testosterone." Testosterone suppresses the immune system, which is another reason why men are so much less likely to get many autoimmune diseases, including MS.

Despite these scientific findings, most doctors miss autoimmune disease in women. Recent studies show that the average woman sees five doctors over four and a half years before receiving a proper diagnosis—and nearly half of patients are labeled as "chronic complainers" in the early stages of their illness.

McCarthy, who researches sex differences in the brain, offers an additional hypothesis as to why women face higher rates of adult chronic conditions including autoimmune disease. "We have good evidence that women are more stressed than men in the modern world," says McCarthy. Girls not only face more adverse experiences when they enter adolescence but also, studies show, are exposed to more interpersonal and other stressors in their day-to-day lives than boys.

Girls are more likely to be criticized for not being attractive or sexy, or for being too sexual, or too fat, or too "flat." Throughout their lives, women are also physically vulnerable, paid less for the same work that men do, and have less career security while carrying more responsibility for child care and caregiving for parents. When women become successful, they are more likely to be seen as aggressive rather than assertive, strident rather than strong.

Girls come of age witnessing these pervasive inequities, and this serves as a chronic stressor that creates wear and tear on the immune system, setting up girls for epigenetic changes and disease. "This idea that girls come of age in a more stressful context doesn't negate any of the other causes we've discussed, but complements them," says McCarthy. "And yet physicians do not take seriously the cost that this societal stress has on the female body."

When women are overtly victimized, this correlation becomes startlingly clear. Bessel van der Kolk, MD, a trauma and recovery psychiatrist and author of *The Body Keeps the Score: Brain, Mind, and Body in the Healing of Trauma,* found that female incest survivors had abnormalities in their ratios of immune cells compared with nontraumatized women. They had a greater proliferation of a particular type of cell that "makes the immune system oversensitive to threats, so that it is prone to mount a defense when none is needed, even when this means attacking the body's own cells," says van der Kolk. This, in turn, puts them more at risk for autoimmune diseases.

A Girl's Brain Is a Vulnerable Brain—in Unique Ways

Ten percent of men with an ACE Score of 1 suffer from chronic depression; 18 percent of women do. Likewise, 33 percent of men with an ACE Score of 4 or more later develop depression—already a high, disturbing figure—while nearly 60 percent of women with that score develop chronic depression in adulthood. The risk that toxic stress will lead to neuroinflammatory diseases such as depression and anxiety disorders is, as with autoimmune disease, nearly twice as high for women as it is for men.

At the University of Wisconsin, neuropsychiatrist Ryan Herringa, MD, PhD, and assistant professor of child and adolescent psychiatry, recently asked a fairly typical group of sixty-four eighteen-year-olds— who were being followed by Herringa's colleagues in a longitudinal study known as the Wisconsin Study of Families and Work—to answer questions about the adversity they'd faced.

They were asked to agree or disagree with statements such as "when I was growing up people called me things like 'stupid,' 'lazy' "; or, "people in my family said hurtful or insulting things to me"; or, "I thought my parents wished I had never been born"; or, "I felt that someone in my family hated me," as well as questions about more overt physical and sexual abuse and emotional neglect.

Then Herringa had the teens undergo MRI brain imaging, in order to measure the connections between three areas of the brain that process and overcome fear.

One of these areas, the prefrontal cortex, helps to analyze thoughts, reflect on them, and decide how to act and behave. You might think of the prefrontal cortex as something like an experience simulator. We try things out in our heads before we actually do them in real life. We can also decide how we feel about a person or place or event that took place in our past, or how we feel about something that's about to happen, like an upcoming lunch with an old boyfriend.

The prefrontal cortex takes its cue on how to process thoughts and reflections from the amygdala, the brain's fear and emotion center—which triggers the fight-or-flight reaction whenever we feel threatened or afraid, or when we remember being in dangerous situations.

The third area of the brain is the hippocampus, which stores memories and helps distinguish false alarms from the real danger signals that the amygdala sends.

As Herringa explains, "If you're at home watching a scary movie at night, the hippocampus can tell the prefrontal cortex that you're at home, this is just a movie, and there is no reason to go into full fight-or-flight response or freak out."

At least that's how these three areas of the brain work together if the brain circuitry that connects them is working correctly. And researchers can see how strong the working connection is through MRI imaging.

Herringa discovered that there was a dramatic difference in the connection between the prefrontal cortex and the hippocampus in both male and female teens who'd suffered adversity, compared with teens who had faced none.

To some degree, that was expected, but these brain changes had occurred even in kids who were experiencing very common, *much milder* forms of childhood adversity in the home, including name calling, teasing, parents who reacted harshly to them, or lack of emotional nurturance.

As a result, "the hippocampus may be having trouble feeding the correct information to the prefrontal cortex about when and where to feel safe, and when not to feel safe, in daily life." This was true even for teenagers who were *not* considered abused, but who had more difficulty differentiating between safe and unsafe environments. This could lead, in turn, to a state of "hypervigilance, of constantly looking around the next corner for the next emotional or physical threat."

Herringa's study provides hard, physical evidence that even mild, low-grade adversity, when chronic, leads to a revved-up alarm system and to inflammation.

For parents, this study's findings may seem worrisome, but we're not talking about the occasional moment when parents are irritated with their kids at the end of a long, stressful workweek or frustrated when the kids won't turn off their computer game to take out the trash. Many parents have had less-than-mindful moments and later regretted being too harsh with a child they love and would never consciously harm. This may be especially true for parents who are already overwhelmed, dealing with health issues, financial stressors, or other problems that are taxing their resources. Or, if they received very little nurturance when they were kids, they may lack the parenting skills to do better with their own kids than their own parents did with them. Often, says Herringa, "this is about parents trying to deal with the harsh events in their own lives, and they don't mean to take it out on their children. They are good parents, doing the best they can with what little they have."

This is not about blame.

But we can use this knowledge about the effect of repeated stress on children we treasure in order to become more mindful parents, coaches, and mentors. (We'll address that directly in Chapter Eight.)

Another surprising finding in Herringa's research was that bad experiences were tied to weaker neural connections between the prefrontal cortex and the hippocampus in the brains of both teenage girls and boys. But neural connections in girls were *also* weaker between the prefrontal cortex and the amygdala, the fear center of the brain itself.

What did this mean? According to Herringa, "This connection between the prefrontal cortex and the amygdala is a direct connection that helps to control our fear and emotional responses." It plays an essential role in determining how emotionally reactive we're likely to be to the things that happen to us in our day-to-day world—and how likely we are to perceive events as stressful or dangerous.

"If you are a girl who has had Adverse Childhood Experiences and these brain connections are weaker, you might expect that in just about any stressful situation you encounter as life goes on—financial stress, a near accident while driving, relationship stress, or family arguments—you may experience a greater level of fear and anxiety in those situations," says Herringa.

Girls with these weakened neural connections are more likely to develop anxiety and depression by the time they reached late adolescence. This correlated with Herringa's observations of young women he'd been following in his clinic for some years. These girls "seemed to be afraid everywhere. It's like they've lost the ability to put a contextual limit on when they're going to be afraid and when they're not." They suffered from fear and anxiety that other teenagers their age who hadn't met with adversity simply were not experiencing.

According to Herringa, maltreatment in childhood impairs the regulatory capacity of the brain's fear circuitry. Moreover, maltreatment's effect on girls' frontal lobe, amygdala, and hippocampal connectivity "may help explain females' higher risk for later having anxiety and depression."

Meanwhile, other researchers have been looking at childhood adversity's effect on the brain through other lenses. Hilary P. Blumberg, MD, professor of psychiatry and director of the Mood Disorders Research Program at Yale School of Medicine, studied forty-two adolescent boys and girls, ages twelve to seventeen, who'd been through childhood trauma and found that there were differences in which areas of the brain were affected depending on the type of adversity they had encountered.

For instance, those who'd experienced physical abuse showed decreases in the prefrontal cortex, as well as in an area of the brain known as the insula cortex. "The insula is associated with having a sense of bodily ownership and personal agency," says Blumberg. These findings suggest that "decreases in this area might be associated with the feelings of disassociation that children who've experienced physical abuse so often report." Kids disassociate from the sense that they are in their own bodies because it's the only way they can escape the terror of what's happening to them. They simply "go elsewhere" mentally—as if it isn't their arm being twisted, or face being slapped, or body being sexually assaulted.

Those children who'd been neglected emotionally showed decreases in areas of the brain that are associated with emotional regulation. Emotional maltreatment, Blumberg says, may "alter the development of the brain circuitry that regulates emotions—in ways that make adolescents more prone to depression."

Blumberg also found striking overall differences in where specific brain changes occurred based on whether a child was male or female. Girls who reported adversity were more likely to experience decreases in gray matter volume in brain regions associated with regulating emotions, and depression—including the prefrontal cortex, amygdala, and hippocampus.

Boys, on the other hand, were more likely to show decreases in brain matter volume in the caudate region of the brain—an area responsible for impulse control and behavior.

Blumberg speculates that the difference in brain changes that occur in girls and boys "might contribute to the relatively greater risk for mood disorders in girls, and disorders of impulse control in boys" who have been exposed to childhood adversity.

Certainly girls can have issues with attention and impulse control, and boys can become depressed and anxious in the aftermath of adversity. Any child psychiatrist can attest to that. Moreover, kids who have never been treated harshly can develop depression, anxiety, and ADHD. Diet, genetics, chemicals, viruses, and infections all play a part. But this recent understanding of the impact of adversity on the brain, and the differences between boys and girls, can help explain some of the adolescent suffering we see.

Ten-year-old Laura's mom faces the loss of her marriage, is depressed and anxious, and criticizes and puts down her daughter regularly. Seven year-old Stephen's dad is under extreme work and financial pressures, and he screams at his son over a flip-flop lost in a lake and calls him "pretty boy." This stress prunes away neurons in the young, developing brain.

Laura and Stephen seem just fine for years; they show no signs of what's happening in their own homes. They smile, do well in school. As they grow into their teen years, however, and their brains go through the normal, developmental pruning process, and neurons are lost, suddenly their brains are functioning at a suboptimal level, shy of the connections needed to create the kind of well-functioning, integrated circuitry to manage mood, suss out danger, and thrive.

Situations that should be everyday moments of complex, messy, but manageable life become hurdles too high. Laura is anxious, reactive, fearful; she has trouble gauging how to properly respond to disagreements small and large. The stressful moments in her day-to-day life blur together; she is always managing a low-grade buzz of anxiety.

As for Stephen, the neural connections between his hippocampus and the prefrontal cortex may be weakened so that he's less able to mentally weigh whether something might be a good decision or not. He may appear indecisive, disorganized. There may be changes, too, in the caudate area of his brain, so that he's less able to control impulsive behavior.

Indeed, research in animal models further illustrates these findings. When researchers induced low states of inflammation into rats' brains in the hippocampus, the animals were no longer able to discern between safe and nonsafe environments. Neuroinflammation disrupted specific neural circuits, leading to impairment in decision making, making it harder to distinguish what was good and what was bad and to make sound choices.

It's a painful way to be in the world.

Girls and the Genetic Link Between Childhood Adversity and Adult Depression

A hormone regulatory gene known as "CRH receptor 1," or the CRHR1 gene—may play a role in protecting some men from depression and anxiety in the face of adversity.

Kerry Ressler, MD, PhD, professor of psychiatry and behavioral sciences at Emory University School of Medicine, is a leading expert on the neurobiology of how fear changes the long-term health of the brain. Even though there is a high correlation between childhood adversity and adult depression, not all individuals who experience childhood trauma develop depression. Women are clearly more vulnerable, but some men—and women—remain resilient even when exposed to stressors in adolescence or adulthood.

Ressler examined the relationship between genetic makeup, the type of abuse, and sex differences that might lead to specific outcomes, and specifically focused on a variant of the CRHR1 gene that he suspected might be protective against the effect of childhood trauma—and the production of stress hormones—which he referred to as protective allele "A."

His team found, as have many studies, that the prevalence of depression was significantly higher among women than in men. They also saw, as Felitti and Anda had, a higher prevalence of women having had fairly high levels of childhood abuse. Forty-four percent of women reported having experienced moderate to severe childhood maltreatment, compared to 35 percent of men. And this difference was almost entirely due to the greater degree to which women had experienced sexual abuse as children. Men, on the other hand, were more likely to have experienced physical abuse as kids.

Ressler recruited more than a thousand subjects from the waiting rooms of a public urban hospital and an urban obstetrical-gynecological clinic and divided them into groups: those who'd suffered emotional abuse, those who'd experienced physical abuse, and those who'd faced sexual abuse. Researchers also subdivided participants into subgroups: those who'd experienced moderate or severe abuse of at least one type and those who'd experienced no abuse at all.

And all three types of maltreatment—emotional, physical, sexual— were significantly correlated with adult depression. But several startling insights emerged that researchers hadn't seen before.

When researchers added in the factor of *gender*, the results were mind-boggling: men with the protective "A" variant of the CRHR1 gene were "significantly protected from developing depression after childhood abuse."

Boys with this gene variant who experience childhood trauma are less likely to develop adult depression, whereas it seemed to make no such difference for women. This is highly significant, Ressler says, "because this is a genetic site that is highly involved in stress regulation," and may play a role in why women have a 2:1 ratio of depression compared with men.

Certainly young men suffer from depression all too frequently— but for some lucky young men, CRHR1 may be a kind of Teflon gene that prevents depression from developing and taking hold after childhood adversity. Other research backs this up. Researchers at the Medical University of South Carolina found that women who had suffered from childhood adversity had higher overall stress-hormone and cortisol responses when they faced a current stressor—in this case, a stress test in the lab—than did men who had a similar history of childhood adversity and had faced the same stressor.

Margaret McCarthy is studying one other sex difference that may affect why women suffer more depression from Adverse Childhood Experiences. She and colleagues have discovered a big sex difference in the growth of new neurons, or neurogenesis, in developing rat pup brains. Males make about twice as many new neurons during the first week of life as females. This is significant, says McCarthy, because making more neurons may allow males to later "forget" some of the bad things that happened to them, including early life adverse events. "Theoretically, this may mean that, as adults, males don't remember their lousy childhood as well as females do, because as they make more neurons, those neurons crowd out old ones and replace them, replacing the memories, as well." If studies bear out this hypothesis, it may give greater insight into why women are affected differently by early adversity.

—

So, here is what we do know: Adversity more often leads to both autoimmune disease and depression in women. Women may carry a biological predisposition to both an increased cortisol response and greater dysregulation of that inflammatory response, following childhood adversity, making us more prone to later health problems in general. Women who have faced childhood adversity show greater disruptions in connections between the areas of the brain that help moderate anxiety and stress reactivity—which in turn leads to a greater chance of depression later in life. And men may have some protective gene variants against developing depression after childhood trauma, but may be more prone to behavior and attention disorders.

Perhaps what is most surprising, given this research, is that even though studies repeatedly show that many girls experience more forms than boys of childhood CUTS, or Chronic Unpredictable Toxic Stress—which affects girls in unique biophysical ways that can lead to depression and autoimmune disease—very few physicians have even a clue that these relationships exist and that they matter.

Vincent Felitti puts it this way. "Every physician will see several patients with high ACE Scores each day. Typically, they are the most difficult patients of the day. More often than not, they are women. And so, all too often, their symptoms, and the underlying causes that play a role both in illness and in healing, will be missed and dismissed."

How extraordinary it is, then, that those 64 percent of Americans—women and men—who have had Adverse Childhood Experiences, nevertheless so often build remarkably loving and decent lives, exhibit such courage and forbearance, and prosper emotionally so much of the time.

CHAPTER FIVE

The Good Enough Family

Parental love is a boon for life. Feeling loved and seen for who we really are, and supported to become who we hope to become, pays forward mentally and physically throughout our lives. Long before the link between childhood adversity and adult health was clear, researchers tried to quantify the benefit of parental love on adult well-being.

In the early 1950s, researchers at Harvard asked 126 healthy male undergraduates to rate their relationship with their mother and father as "very close," "tolerant," or "strained and cold" in order to get a sense of the students' perceptions of how loving, fair, just, and kind their parents had been to them.

Thirty-five years later, in 1993, psychologists took a look at the medical records of the men, who were now in their fifties and sixties. Ninety-one percent of men who, decades earlier, had cited their relationship with Mom as "tolerant" or "strained and cold," had been diagnosed with some form of serious illness by the time they hit midlife, including heart disease, high blood pressure, and ulcers. One hundred percent of students—every single one—who said their relationship with *both* of their parents was "strained and cold," or "tolerant," developed serious diseases by middle age.

Only 45 percent of those who'd described their relationships with their mom as "warm and friendly" developed disease by their fifties. The young men who felt loved by Dad also faced less illness in midlife.

So researchers ran the numbers another way, looking at specific words that the young people chose to describe their parents. Ninety-five percent of those who *didn't* describe Mom and Dad in a positive light later developed heart disease, hypertension, and other diseases. This was true regardless of family medical history, whether or not they smoked, were divorced, or their parents had died or were divorced.

Researchers at Johns Hopkins ran a similar study, looking at the relationship of male medical students with their parents and their health forty and fifty years later. Students with less warm and loving relationships were far more likely to develop cancer in midlife.

The Harvard and Johns Hopkins researchers concluded that no other single factor was more significantly related to illness than the degree of parental closeness one enjoyed growing up. In fact, lack of parental closeness was a more significant contributor to later disease than smoking, drinking, parental divorce, having a parent die, or being exposed to harmful, toxic environmental substances.

When You Hope to Be a Better Parent than Your Parents Were

As Stanford neuroscientist and MacArthur fellow Robert Sapolsky recently tweeted: "There's nothing like parenthood to make you really neurotic as you worry about the consequences of your every act, thought, or omission."

Many individuals who grew up with Adverse Childhood Experiences later worry about what kind of parent they will be.

Cindy grew up as the eighth child in a large Catholic family that was always chaotic.

Cindy's mother, who grew up in an alcoholic family, began having children at nineteen. By the time Cindy was born, two months premature, her oldest sister was a teenager. By then, Cindy says, "My mom had been raising kids for more than sixteen years."

"Growing up, I felt my mother was almost like a kind of war victim," Cindy tells me. "I've been told that because I was premature, I got more attention when I was born than my siblings did. I had that, at least, on my side."

Weak parenting skills were passed down on both sides of Cindy's family tree. Cindy's grandmother was widowed very young and raised Cindy's father and his five brothers with an iron fist. "And so he ruled us with the iron fist he'd inherited from her," she says.

Cindy's parents divorced when she was young. Her father left. Then, when she was twelve, Cindy's mother announced, "I've been parenting for thirty years and I want to be on my own. Go live with your father. Let him deal with it all." Her dad's new wife didn't like spending money on her husband's kids and "complained about the price of our dentist bills.

"I was really good in school, and my dad valued that, so in some ways I walked on water with my dad," Cindy says. A wan smile crosses her face. "That saved me. My father was very achievement-oriented and rewarded me for doing well but he was always pushing. If I got an A he'd say, 'Why wasn't it an A+?' My good grades became a double-edged sword and he'd say, 'You think you're so book smart, but you have no common sense!' And that just wasn't true."

But those moments of shame were minuscule compared "to what he did to my brother," Cindy says. "He never lifted a hand to me, but he was really brutal to my brother who was only nine when my parents divorced." Cindy says she has "a vivid memory of one day when he was about eleven, my brother was on the floor and my father was just beating him in front of me. My brother would punch holes in the wall in our house. He was so angry and hurt. My father's approach was to control with force, while my mother was just overwhelmed by it all. And my father never took responsibility for how he damaged him." Cindy's brother went to college for a little while and then dropped out.

Another brother went to college, then eventually started a deck construction company. "I remember my dad telling him, 'I'm embarrassed to tell people you're my son; all you do is pound nails for a living.'"

"I watched my siblings suffer," she says. "One sister ended up in a group home in her twenties after my parents told her she had to move out. Another developed serious addictions. I was a bystander to all of that, too." Cindy recalls having "this aha moment" from the age of ten or eleven, "this internal dialogue with myself that if I want to get out of here, I will have to *achieve* my way out. Doing well on every test, every paper, felt like a matter of sheer survival. I was plotting my escape from a very early age." And her strategy worked. She graduated from a well-known liberal arts college.

By age twenty, however, Cindy's immune system started breaking down. "I started coming down with every flu and cold around," she says. "One infection morphed into the next. For about a year I was almost never well." I developed chronic urinary tract problems, which led to "this terrible phobia about having to urinate. It was a very self-reinforcing cycle where worry and anxiety made my urinary tract symptoms far worse. It was as if my immune system was so tired of doing battle."

Then Cindy developed acute muscle pain. "One day, in my early twenties, my neck hurt so badly—without my even knowing how I had hurt it—that I couldn't lift my head to get out of bed." Altered immune function, increased risk of infection, muscle spasms, and pain—she was twentysomething but had an old woman's excruciatingly painful and worn-out body.

Cindy worked hard at building her career and searched, in a remarkably conscious and careful way, for someone she could love and be loved by who was very different from her father. "Someone who wasn't critical, someone who listened, someone who saw the best in people." Cindy met her husband when she was only twenty-four. "I felt this huge window of healing open up for me; he was this stable presence I'd long needed in my life."

But as her life became more stable, she slowly became more aware of her own emotional unsteadiness. "Some nights I'd have panic attacks and my husband would spend hours just listening and talking me down." At a certain point, "I recognized how unfair that was to him. I told him, 'I could cry on your shoulder forevermore, but I need to grow up so I can be a full partner. I don't want to be the broken one. And at some point you are going to get weary from always being the listener, the strong one.'"

Cindy worried so much about what kind of parent she might be that she didn't see how she could ever have kids. "I was so afraid of not having the skills to parent, and of passing on the pain of my childhood. I knew there had to be a better way to live than how I had been raised. I knew that life shouldn't be so painful."

Cindy understood how deeply her past was affecting her and told her husband, "I will not have children until I know that I am in an emotionally stable place and can give them what any child deserves."

Cindy and her husband had their first son when Cindy was in her early thirties. "We both cut back on our work hours; we were tag-team parents all the way." Cindy loved her work, and her son was a happy baby, which gave her the confidence to have a second child at the age of thirty-five. Her second child, a girl, was a far more challenging baby.

"She was one of those babies who could not be comforted," Cindy says. "At times she would cry, scream at the top of her lungs." Her daughter was highly sensitive to stimuli, reactive to loud noises, unsettled. Cindy felt anxious when she couldn't help her to stop crying. "I felt inside that I was failing as a mom. Because I had no template for what it meant to be a good parent, I didn't know what normal was," Cindy says. "So I became this whirling dervish trying to be the perfect, loving, always attentive parent, without thinking enough about my own well-being. On the rare occasions when my daughter would nap, I would push myself to spend more time playing with my preschooler."

As her daughter got older and more settled, life got easier. "That is, until perimenopause hit." Cindy's physical and emotional symptoms returned. The depression she had wrestled with when she was younger came back, as did panic attacks. She was engulfed by a flulike fatigue. She felt less able to manage her emotions. She started a new job she was excited about, but it didn't work out as she'd hoped. She forgot things, then felt ashamed.

The saying "Fear swallows children—and the adults we become" was true for Cindy. "After years of having felt more capable of handling whatever came along, I'd wake up thrashing in the middle of the night. I blamed myself for not being able to will myself to handle life better. If we've had a difficult childhood, years later all the events of our past begin to seem surreal. It's as if they never really happened, so we forget the impact they've had on us. I felt that if my childhood wasn't happening to me right now, why should it still be impacting me so much? Why couldn't I just move on? The combination of perimenopause and work stress reignited the trauma from my childhood. It brought up emotional challenges that I hadn't struggled with for a long time."

Cindy recognized that she needed to find ways to heal herself if she hoped to keep the past of "my own childhood from spilling into my children's present-day lives."

The Reactive Parent

Grace also worries about her childhood's influence on her parenting of her own children.

Grace has five-year-old twin girls and woke up seemingly overnight to a diagnosis of multiple sclerosis at forty-one. When she was growing up, her younger sister had leukemia, and died when Grace was twelve. Grace was her bone marrow donor.

Grace says it's hard to provide even-keeled parenting, given that in her own childhood world, "The other shoe just kept dropping. You worried every day, 'What's coming next? Will my parents be home tonight, or at the hospital? Will my baby sister be alive tomorrow?' I think that probably gave me a very different nervous system than if I'd had a family life in which the four of us sailed through. All my parents could think about was my sister, and I understood that. Our parents were great parents, but they couldn't really be my parents and give my sister all that she needed and deserved at the same time.

"When I was pregnant, all I could think of was, Will my twins be born healthy? Will I survive delivery? But my friends who were pregnant around the same time were not stressing in that way. They were searching online for onesies with cute logos on them.

"I'm always on the worst-case-scenario channel in my mind," Grace admits. "I was with the girls at our local playground. One of my daughters ran up to me and said, 'That boy was mean, Mommy, he called me a bad name!' She was sobbing. And seeing her that way made *me* so upset, I was shaking instantaneously. Literally my hands were shaking, my fingers jumping around. I just could not speak calmly. I was so upset about how devastated and lost my daughter seemed. Before I could think about it, I took both my girls by the hand and yelled to this boy's mother, "You need to do something about your son—he's a bully!" I began walking home, pulling them along, and they were both crying. My mind was just buzzing as I replayed the whole scene. I was so preoccupied I didn't bother to soothe *them*. I just dragged them along while I mentally rehashed what I should have said or done differently.

"I don't want to parent like this," Grace says. "I don't want to be that kind of mom who is so caught up in her own anxiety she can't think about what's best for her kids in a calm, cogent, reassuring way. How can you soothe your kids with shaking hands?" Grace wants to teach her kids by example how to deal with life mindfully, calmly: "I want to be the kind of mom who, even if the house were on fire, could get my kids out, then sit with my arms around them on the curb as firemen put out the flames, and say, 'It's all going to be okay, everything is going to be all right.' But that calm mom is the opposite of who I am."

For someone else, with a different set of Adverse Childhood Experiences—for instance, with parents who had ridiculed and diminished her when she was needy—the reaction might be the opposite of Grace's. She might shut down her own feelings and those of her children, underreact, and tell her child to forget about it: "Don't be sad, don't cry, go back in there and play!" Or, she might lace her comments with criticism, "Don't be a crybaby!"

Either way, whether parents overreact or underreact, a toddler gets the message, When I feel bad and tell Mommy, I just make Mommy feel sadder—or madder; *Mommy can't help me.*

As Grace puts it, "I know I am not the mom I want to be. I'm trying, but I'm not there yet. I sometimes beat myself up for that. I wonder, what *is* the good enough mom?'"

———

Parenting is simply the hardest, best job you'll ever have. As a parent, you want your kids to know that you will offer them welcome arms, a safe haven, no matter what occurs. We always want our kids to feel that same sense of love we gave them when they were small, and came running into our arms. "*There you are, there you are,*" we tell them. They know they are what matters most to us in all the world.

But parenting mindfully and taking care of all of your children's needs amid life's challenges is demanding. Sometimes there is simply too much to navigate or we're exhausted. Kids can be uncooperative and endlessly energetic. Teens can be self-centered, flippant, forgetful, defiant, and make poor choices. It's easy to be overwhelmed, lose your patience, and mutter or yell things you regret. If you are parenting teenagers, you almost certainly will lose it now and then.

Not every experience in family life can be "loving and close," "warm and friendly," or "understanding and sympathetic." Family glitches happen—one person's reactivity ignites another's meltdown. (I have a friend who refers to family meltdowns this way: "It was not our *best* day as a family.")

We never know what small comments—words that are less than skillful or wise but are nonetheless not messages that foster childhood adversity—will be misunderstood or misinterpreted, stick in our kid's head, and bounce around in there for years, causing resentments we don't even know about.

We parent in the moment, as best we can. When we fall short, we hope that our shortfalls will be forgotten.

Yet the Adverse Childhood Experiences Survey and Childhood Trauma Questionnaire tell us that only about one-third of kids grow up in families in which no ACEs occur. That means that nearly two-thirds of parents are struggling in some way, whether they know it or not. Maybe their stressors stem from events, illnesses, outside influences, accidents, or losses beyond their control.

For our purposes, however, we're going to look at the latest neuroscientific findings on how your own childhood Chronic Unpredictable Toxic Stress might affect your ability to parent as well as you'd like. It's important to step back and ask yourself, with absolute honesty, how reactive am I in my family life?

Happily, even if the answer is "very," it's not too late for us, or for our children.

It's Hard to Give What Your Brain Never Received

There is a saying that you learn how to love others through the love others show you—but what if no one showed you how? Recent findings from interpersonal biology show that early losses and chronic unpredictable stress alter the neurocircuitry of the young brain in ways that dramatically change our later ability to create and nurture successful, meaningful relationships.

The work of Robin Karr-Morse, family therapist and coauthor of *Ghosts from the Nursery: Tracing the Roots of Violence*, reveals that trauma experienced prenatally and in the first three years of life can make us more likely to be reactive as a parent, partner, or spouse.

"Although the brain develops throughout childhood and the teen years, the environment in the womb and during the first three years of life is a critical period during which the fundamental structure and chemistry of the brain are set in place," says Karr-Morse.

For instance, when a baby perceives any threat through her senses, such as loud, angry voices in the next room, her brain goes on alert. Baby's heart pumps, her breath becomes rapid and shallow, she sweats, and oxygen rushes to her limbs in an involuntary fight-or-flight response. But since a baby can neither fight nor flee, "she will move into a third neurological state, known as a 'freeze' state," says Karr Morse. Baby doesn't cry or scream but goes sort of numb. This freeze state is a trauma state.

"In a brand-new little nervous system," Karr-Morse says, "it doesn't take a lot to put a baby into trauma. When this kind of emotional trauma happens routinely, a tiny baby can spend a great deal of time in this freeze state."

Once the brain has become hypervigilant to danger, it is more easily triggered: the amygdala stays on high alert to assess what's coming next. And whenever it detects danger signals in the baby's environment, that little brain quickly goes into a heightened state of vigilance.

Researchers call this phenomenon "kindling." Now it takes only a tiny spark, a small trigger, for the baby's brain to burst into a firestorm of reactivity, releasing a sudden blaze of stress hormones and chemicals. Exposure to early stress is like laying kindling in the brain so that, says Karr-Morse, "a person who has had early chronic trauma is much more susceptible to later reactivity to stressful events."

This process can begin prenatally. "It's common for women in pregnancy to be stressed, but to be extremely stressed chronically, where the mother's HPA axis is already chronically on fight or flight, means that that baby is growing in an environment that is bathing in far too much cortisol," she explains. "And that can have a tremendous influence on the nervous system of the fetus, so that the baby, from birth, might be susceptible or hypervigilant or vulnerable to any form of stimulation, because their nervous system is set on high."

If a new mom has postpartum depression, or is neglectful, or overreactive, that will further impede the "baby learning to regulate his or her own nervous system."

Unavoidable events, such as hospitalization in neonatal intensive care, can also set the developing nervous system on high.

A mom's physical health during pregnancy can also affect her child's lifelong health. If Mom has a flu during certain windows of pregnancy, that viral impact makes it more likely that her child will develop schizophrenia or autism. Similarly, babies who were conceived during years of famine, and received poor nutrition in the womb, grow up to have more health problems and are smaller in adulthood—whereas babies whose pregnant moms are well fed grow up to be healthier and physically bigger. These effects can last for generations, affecting grandchildren's health as well. This research helps us to better understand how the prenatal stressors our mother may have faced can influence both our physical and emotional well-being in long-lasting ways.

How Children Absorb Their Parents' Stress

Researchers have been examining other ways in which parental stress can be passed on from parent to child. Some of their findings are surprising. Scientists at the University of Haifa have found, for instance, that children may even inherit the effects of a mother's stress from events that occurred before conception through their DNA.

Mildly stressed female lab rats who were mated with nonstressed male rats had offspring that showed more anxiety than babies born to nonstressed mothers. Stressed female rats showed an increased expression of a particular protein that prompted cells to release *more* hormones related to stress and anxiety. The more this protein was expressed, the more stressed the female rat became, and the more stressed her babies were. Even more startling, this anxious behavior was passed along from a mom to her offspring epigenetically—the stress had nothing to do with the later quality of parental care: this stress protein *already existed* in large concentrations in the eggs of these previously stressed females—before the mom rats became pregnant.

This suggests that a female's eggs were transferring "soft-wired information." In other words, Mom's eggs were transmitting Mom's trauma to her babies before they were born.

All this research has been done on rats, and not humans, since we can't take out parts of the human brain, slice them up, and study them. But it gives support to the idea that stress may be transferred from a mother's cells to her child in ways we are only beginning to understand.

Stress can also be transmitted between parent and child through what researchers call "empathic stress." Studies show that merely observing another person in a stressful situation can trigger a physical stress response in you. If you're with someone who's stressed out, their stress can become your stress, not just emotionally, but biologically: your cortisol levels rise along with theirs. This is "empathetic stress."

Stress can affect infants, in the same way, through what's known as "contagious emotions." Researchers at the University of California, San Francisco (UCSF), set out to determine how this happens between mother and child. "Our earliest lessons about how to manage stress and strong negative emotions in our day-to-day lives occur in the parent-child relationship," says Sara Waters, a lead researcher in the study. And it appears that this transmission goes far beyond words or even visible expressions.

Waters and her colleagues recruited sixty-nine mothers and their twelve- to fourteen-month-old infants. They hooked up mothers and children to cardiovascular sensors and took baseline readings when moms and infants were sitting and resting together. Then, they separated mothers from their babies and asked them to deliver a prepared five-minute speech to evaluators—then answer evaluators' questions for another five minutes.

A third of the mothers were treated quite positively by evaluators, who listened, nodding their heads, smiling as these moms spoke, leaning forward as if to ferret out more. Another third of the moms received negative feedback; evaluators frowned, shook their heads, and crossed their arms as if they didn't like what they were hearing. And another third of the moms didn't interact with evaluators at all.

Afterward, the moms who received negative feedback showed increased cardiac stress and admitted they had more negative feelings than positive ones.

Researchers then reunited babies with their moms.

Those infants who were placed back in the arms of moms whose talks had been reviewed negatively by evaluators picked up on their mothers' emotional distress right away. The greater a mom's physiological stress, the greater her infant's physiological stress response was once the child was back in the mother's arms. These infants' heart rates went up—spiking higher than they had been at baseline—within moments of being reunited with their stressed-out moms.

These babies couldn't talk and express what they were sensing. They just knew something was off. Mommy was stressed. And so were they.

These infants, says Waters, "caught the psychological residue of their mother's stressful experiences." She explains: "We may overlook how exquisitely attuned babies are to the emotional tenor of their caregivers before they are verbal and able to fully express themselves." An infant "may not be able to tell you that you seem stressed, or ask you what's wrong, but as soon as she is in your arms, she is picking up on the bodily responses that accompany your emotional state— transmitted through vocal tension, heart rate, facial expressions, odor, or other difficult-to-see mother-to-child avenues of 'stress contagion.'" In this way, an infant may silently absorb her parents' negative emotions into her own tiny body.

Parental conflict—which often increases when new parents are coping with the stress of sleepless nights, new schedules, less time to devote to their relationship, and perhaps differing views over what's best for baby—can also affect how reactive an infant's brain is to stress.

Research shows that babies can also pick up on and absorb the stress of parental bickering—including when the baby is sleeping. Oregon Health and Science University researcher Alice Graham, PhD, discovered this when she asked mothers to fill out surveys on how often they tended to argue with their partners at home, and then examined the brain activity of their six- to twelve-month-olds with functional magnetic resonance imaging, or fMRI.

Graham's team put headphones on these babies while they were sleeping during the fMRI scan, and played nonsense phrases read in both neutral and angry voices. Babies whose parents argued a lot at home showed a stronger neurological reaction when they heard angry tones in areas of the brain that are associated with processing stress and emotion.

Parental Stress Translates into a Child's Pain

Parental stress can affect children's physical health as they grow and develop. For instance, kids whose moms suffer from anxiety and depression are far more likely to develop physical symptoms—including headaches, stomachaches, pain, and fatigue—by the time they turn five, six, and seven years old. This may be, at least in part, because depressed moms often react to their children's emotional needs differently than nondepressed moms do.

Because Grace, for instance, was so caught up in her own emotions—to the point that they built up and spilled over into an angry overreaction—her three-year-old twin daughters didn't get the soothing they needed. Nor did they learn from Grace how to self-regulate their own distress.

In one recent study, mothers from a range of racial and socioeconomic backgrounds who had either come to terms with their early negative experiences or who had had positive experiences with their own caregivers were better able to respond to their newborn infants' cries and comfort them. Conversely, depressed moms or those who still had difficulty controlling their emotions regarding the past exhibited more rapid heart rates, showed greater signs of distress as measured by the amount of sweat on their skin—and they were less able to respond to their babies' crying. Instead these moms were more focused on themselves than on the needs of their distressed baby.

When a child does not get help in regulating his anxiety and stays in fight-or-flight mode, he's far more likely to develop physical symptoms that will persist through his childhood and teenage years into adulthood. Toddlers whose moms can't soothe them are more likely to be obese or develop metabolic syndrome by the time they are teens. These teens who didn't learn to calm themselves may latch on to less-healthy self-soothing: staying up late, watching TV to assuage anxiety and insomnia, and overeating or eating junk food.

Other studies of mothers and children in lower socioeconomic groups not included in the original ACE Study show that many mid-life health problems, including metabolic syndrome, can be traced back to what happened in early childhood. The good news is that kids who have a nurturing mother do better—even when they have fewer economic advantages. Children whose parents showed concern for their welfare, and helped them learn how to cope with stress, were healthier than other kids. In fact, a nurturing mother offsets the metabolic consequences of childhood disadvantage.

Nonparental Stressors: School and Friends

Other key relationships that can positively and negatively influence a child and his development include siblings, friends, coaches, and teachers. A child's experiences during the long hours he spends at school, and with his peers, also affect his stress pathways. Indeed, being excluded or bullied by peers can lead to lifelong health consequences.

John, now forty years old, suffers from major gut problems and chronic fatigue. He understands the relationship between his struggles with his narcissistic dad and his adult health problems. But, he points out, there is "no box to check" on the Adverse Childhood Experiences Survey for "the bullying I faced when I was young."

In seventh grade, John says, "It was the worst. We moved to California from across the country. And this kid at my new school started picking on me, telling me I had a 'really big head.' As in a physically *big* head. Then he got two other kids in on it and the three of them would sit in a ring of seats around me in every class. They'd tease me and pick on me whenever they could get away with it." By eighth grade it got worse. The boys took his stuff. One day, in science class, John says, "This same boy stole my backpack right before it was time to turn in our homework. I just couldn't take it anymore. I was just so tired of getting bullied. I started to get my backpack back from this kid and we got in this tug-of-war, struggling, each holding a strap, when one strap broke and he fell down. He told the teacher and his parents that I pushed him and my dad got really upset with me. My mom had my back, and she believed me. But my dad did not take up my side."

Bullying is a form of adversity linked to illnesses and disease in adulthood. Investigators at Duke recently followed 1,420 boys and girls between the ages of nine and twenty-one who had been victims of bullying—as well as the kids who bullied them. They regularly tested these kids' blood levels of C-reactive protein, or CRP, a marker of systemic inflammation that physicians look at to help diagnose cardiovascular and other diseases. The victims of bullying had higher CRP levels, which rose in direct relationship to the number of bullying events they'd endured.

"The only other kind of social adversity where we see this kind of long-term effect is in children who are physically abused or neglected," says William E. Copeland, associate professor of psychiatry at Duke and one of the authors of the study. "This kind of social defeat is more potent and long-lasting than we previously thought."

Other studies show that children who experience bullying are much more likely to later suffer from depression, anxiety, and other mental health disorders. When kids struggle with the overall pain of social exclusion in their peer relationships, that social pain hurts physically. Brain scans show this to be true. Social pain, the kind that occurs if, say, a child is repeatedly excluded during every game, activates the same brain circuits that are associated with the sensory processing of physical pain.

In one study, which followed eight hundred kids from the age of sixteen to forty-three, adolescents whose teachers had reported that they had problematic peer relationships later had a far higher likelihood of developing cardiovascular disease, high blood pressure, and obesity in middle age. This occurred whether or not they had also had adversity in the home.

This is particularly troubling considering recent stats that show bullying is prevalent. A recent SAFE survey found that about one in four schoolchildren in the United States is bullied regularly during school hours. Kids in grades six through ten are the most likely to be victims of bullies and to join in bullying. Almost half of all kids reported fearing harassment or bullying in the bathroom at school, and many kids who said they'd faced bullying made excuses or tried to find ways to avoid going to school.

Bullying now extends past the schoolyard and into the home. Bullies can find a kid with a smartphone wherever he or she goes, anytime. Disturbingly, about 80 percent of all high school students have been bullied online, and about 15 percent say they've been threatened online.

Trouble at home and trouble at school are often related. Christina Bethell, PhD, professor at the Bloomberg School of Public Health at Johns Hopkins, found that 48 percent of children from birth to age seventeen have experienced one of nine types of Adverse Childhood Experiences, and 23 percent experienced two or more. Children exposed to at least two ACEs were more than two and a half times more likely to repeat a grade, or to be disengaged with their classwork, compared to those who had no such experiences. After accounting for differences in a child's age, race, and income, those with two or more ACEs were nearly five times more likely to have some type of emotional, behavioral, or developmental problem such as ADHD, anxiety, or depression. Specifically, they were over three times more likely to have ADHD. And more than three-quarters of children who had emotional, behavioral, or developmental problems such as ADHD, anxiety, or depression had experienced ACEs.

Other studies have shown that children with a single ACE Score are ten times more likely to have learning and behavior problems compared with those not exposed to trauma, chronic unpredictable stress, or neglect. And those with Adverse Childhood Experiences are thirty times more likely to have behavior or learning problems than those not exposed to childhood adversity. Teachers may suggest that these children be treated for ADHD, not knowing that they need treatment for trauma or PTSD, which involves psychotherapy. The symptoms are the same, but the treatments are entirely different.

The chronic worry and anxiety kids feel about doing well and performing at school and the race to get into college itself can also be a major life stressor.

Vicki Abeles, documentarist of *Race to Nowhere*, raises awareness about the potential long-term impact of unhealthy school stress, how this chronic stress is linked to alarming rises in teenage anxiety, sleeplessness, and depression, and what we can do about it. She believes our achievement-obsessed culture is creating a new form of childhood adversity that's gone unnoted and untreated.

"It's plain to see the harm that our achievement-obsessed culture is doing to kids," she says. "Teens nationwide are routinely grinding through twelve-hour days of school, sports, and homework, striving to reach society's impossible image of success." Abeles believes this "high-stakes grind in school throughout the formative and fragile teen years leads, like every form of childhood adversity, to a stew of stress hormones flooding our kids' still-growing brain and body— setting teens up for a lifetime cycle of anxiety and depression, weakening their immune systems, and making them far more vulnerable to infections and cardiovascular disease for the rest of their lives." Kids are facing excessive societal pressure to perform during the teenage years; they're caught up in this crazy modern race to get the grades to get into a top college—and are overwhelmed with the fear of failure if they don't, Abeles says. "They are ticking time bombs for later ill health."

Recently, the American Psychological Association released a nationwide survey called Stress in America, which found that American teens now report that their stress level during the school year is nearly 6 on a 10-point scale—a level considered emotionally unhealthy, and far higher than that cited by most adults. In this survey of more than one thousand teenagers ages thirteen to seventeen, many teens reported being overwhelmed or depressed because of stress. Eighty-three percent of teens said that school was "a somewhat or significant source of stress." More than one in four reported "extreme stress" during the school year. Forty percent of teens reported feeling angry or irritable during the prior month of school. Almost one in three said stress made them feel as though they could cry.

In summer, stress levels dropped strikingly.

Many kids are so anxious about measuring up that doing well involves far more than learning to grind through the kind of normative stress that is a given in growing up—coping on a bad day when they get a disappointing grade, or getting through a really tough week when exams or SATs loom. The stress response stays activated for prolonged periods of time—in many cases, from September to June. That's chronic stress.

Think of how researchers induce a high-stress state in lab settings. They ask study participants to do math problems or give a short speech—while researchers evaluate them—perfectly mimicking school stress. In other words, researchers re-create a stressful school-like environment to get individuals' cortisol responses to spike. Our high school and college admissions systems may be turning high school into a potentially toxic laboratory, where students' heart rates, blood pressure, blood sugar, stress hormone levels, and immune systems are too often activated.

Yes, for short periods—like when taking an exam—that's good, it helps a young person experience that sense of urgency to get through it and do his utmost best. But when it's a day-in and day-out state of being, when it becomes "the way life is" for students, chronic stress will disrupt brain architecture, cause epigenetic changes and a greater stress response, inflammation, ailments, depression, and disease. It will also disrupt the brain circuitry that plays a role in learning and achieving academic success. When the amygdala is always in a red alert state— *What happens if I don't perform well enough on this test? Will any college want me?*—it's harder to do well. It's not surprising that, in the past decade, rates of "test anxiety" have risen, along with rising teen stress rates and rates of chronic pain and illness, including migraine syndromes and back pain. No wonder many competitive public and private schools are dubbed "stress mills." We might think of many teens' school stress today as "adverse academic experiences."

By the time teens enter college, even those from that one-third of happy-family homes, they may have become accustomed to day-to-day pressures that precipitate an amygdala-reactive stress state that will shadow them throughout their academic and work careers. For those who face their share of adversity at home, there may suddenly be no safe haven.

More tests, more pressure in school and in sports and in the race to get into a good college—more chronic unpredictable stress—and on little sleep: this is not a recipe for being resilient, or developing grit, or building up the brain. It's a recipe for breaking down the brain.

It doesn't really matter what the stressor is, whether it's poverty or chronic abuse or the bully on the bus—stress impacts how the structure and architecture of the brain form.

Early Biology Affects Later Relationships

Recently, after another long-term romantic relationship disintegrated, John grew more curious about the role his Adverse Childhood Experiences played in his poor health and relationship problems. He saw patterns and fundamental insecurities in his behavior that he couldn't shake, which seemed rooted in childhood experiences. He says, "That was a catalyst to look more deeply at how my past is driving my present."

John recalls that when he was in college, and later pursuing a PhD, "my dad never asked me what I was doing, what I was studying; he never asked about my career at all. He would just tell me about what he thought I didn't know." A few years later, John was working for a well-known think tank in New York. John's parents and sister were visiting, and John was asked, on short notice, to speak to a large audience about a project he'd managed and share what had inspired his work. His parents and sister watched John give an hour-long talk about his interests and passions. "I realized afterward that everything I'd said that day in a public forum, about what drives me, were things I'd never said to my own father in any way, shape, or form." Afterward, "My mom said, 'I loved it! It was so great to hear your story. You were wonderful!' My dad stood next to her and said absolutely nothing. Not a word. In that moment, he could not offer me a single word of praise."

And this "lack of respect or love for who I am, this sense that I have no worth," John says, "permeated the nature of our relationship."

Recently, John's parents needed a new car. He told his dad, "I'll give you the money, let's get this done." John bought his dad the car, and on the way home, John was pulling into his parents' garage when his dad started telling him how poorly he was positioning the car. "And I flipped my shit," John says. "I started screaming at him, and even as I was screaming I was so upset with myself for losing it, because I didn't want to be that reactive person. I didn't want to be that way. I didn't want to be him."

John says he lives with an inner whisper of unworthiness, of "never feeling that I could be loved as I am. And that feeling has followed me into all of my relationships in insidious ways. I have such depths of insecurity."

He believes that this same whisper of unworthiness is what causes him to flail in relationships. "The thing I want most is to be comfortable with myself and happy in the world, but each time I come close to having a strong relationship, I sabotage it," John says. "I am so damaged, and so uncomfortable in my own skin, that I don't know how to be with someone who is comfortable in their own skin. And so in order to get away from that discomfort, from the way in which I don't fit into the world, I cut myself off from the thing that I want most: love."

He recalls that when, in his early thirties, he walked out on the girlfriend he so deeply loved, he beat himself up "ten ways to Sunday." He was in so much grief at the recognition of what he'd done, he says, "I lost ten pounds. I couldn't eat. I was still in grad school and I would drive off this bridge on the way to work and think, 'What if I just drive myself off this bridge? I don't deserve to live anyway.'"

In recent relationships, John has found himself behaving more "needy than I would like, while remaining distant and critical. I latch on, and need someone to tell me that I am okay even as I push that person away. I have internalized my dad's voice of shame and blame, only now I am the one who is feeding my inner critic. I can't get free of that low whisper of inadequacy, so I want someone else to free me, to tell me I am lovable."

This past year, at forty, John decided to seek help. "As I told my therapist how badly I wanted a long-term relationship with someone, I just broke down and cried," he says. "I had this feeling that I just could not ever achieve that."

John recognizes that "that spark of life that every kid has, that their parents encourage in them, that reassures them that they are good and right in the world, my dad had tried to extinguish that in me because he didn't feel that in himself."

This shame John feels is not his shame. It comes from having been raised by a narcissist father, which makes it hard for him to believe that he can be loved or wanted, so he tends to react as if he is unwanted. Because he had a parent whom he couldn't trust or get close to, he has trouble understanding the language of love and intimacy.

Over time, emotional volatility and stress reactivity lead to physical pain and relationship pain.

But there is something else at play here, too. Childhood adversity creates profound functional changes in areas of the brain that govern how we recognize our own feelings, voice what we need and want, and empathize with other people. These are all skills that we—and someone like John—need in order to connect with other people and have thriving relationships.

The Neurobiology of Love

Ruth Lanius, MD, PhD, is a neuroscientist and professor of psychiatry and director of the post-traumatic stress disorder (PTSD) research unit at the University of Western Ontario in Canada. She has spent her academic career looking at how neurological changes to a young brain from trauma and adversity affect the ability to interrelate with others over a lifetime.

When our brain is at rest, when nothing major is going on—when, say, we're in between intense feeling states—it is in a state of "idling," says Lanius. When the brain is idling, a network of neurocircuitry known as the brain's "default mode network" quietly hums along, like a car idling in the driveway. Areas of the brain in the default mode network include those associated with memory, those that help us to construct thought, to recognize that others have thoughts, and to help us to integrate our thoughts. All of these regions are integral to our internal thought process.

This network is always on standby, ready to help us figure out what we need to do next. "The dense connectivity in these areas of the brain help us to determine what's relevant or not relevant, so that we can be ready for whatever our environment is going to ask of us," says Lanius. "It is also integrally connected to areas of the brain that relate to one's sense of self, one's feeling state."

People who have suffered trauma have very little connectivity in the default mode network. Their basic sense of self, of who they are at the core, when at rest or at peace, is very weak. The brain seems not to have a healthy idling position—or, to put it another way, a sense of equilibrium. Even milder trauma, Lanius says—the unpredictable chronic stressors of Adverse Childhood Experiences—can hurt the neuroconnectivity in this part of the brain. "It is very moving to see on brain scans what happens when this default mode network is not working well in people. In some sense you might say that when there is little connectivity in the default mode network, people lack what we think of as a sense of self."

Damage to the default network in the brain occurs after repeated trauma creates a sense of powerlessness. Children can't escape from home or their tormentors, and can't flee or fight, so they freeze in place instead. They become emotionally immobilized.

Child psychiatrist Dan Siegel, MD, author of *Brainstorm: The Power and Purpose of the Teenage Brain*, and a scientific leader in interpersonal biology, explains a child's dilemma this way. "When a parent is the source of trauma, a child's brain says, Run from this person to survive. But at the same time, the brain also says, Run to this person—they *are* my survival.

"If one part of the brain says 'Go to Mom,' and the brain stem says, 'Go away,' it's an unsolvable biological paradox," says Siegel. "Two circuits in the brain are activated with completely different goals. A child cannot do both at the same time. The mind of the child fragments because those two circuits are trying to function together and integrate, and they can't."

Parents who can't manage their own feelings and reactions can be terrifying to kids. They're a chronic, unpredictable stressor in their children's lives. To the children, "Emotions become futile," says Lanius. "It would drive you crazy to be feeling a lot of emotions and yet to know you can't act on what you feel, and so you become disassociated from your feeling state, you become emotionally unaware of what's going on around you."

Even if the trauma emanates from another source of adversity—a parent has died, or is deathly ill, or a child's parents are divorcing—a child can't resolve their fight-or-flight reaction by fighting or fleeing. It's just not going to help.

The default-mode network, Lanius says, starts to go offline. It's no longer helping that child to figure out what's relevant, or what he needs to be aware of in order to figure out what to do next. "Shutting down one's feelings becomes the only way to survive childhood," says Lanius. Which means that people with chronic early life trauma often emerge from childhood very unaware of their feeling states.

Years later, this freezing or shutting off has immense consequences in relationships. We may simply turn off unpleasant feelings, unable to respond with compassion for ourselves or others, or be turned off by anyone showing signs of neediness in general. We might not recognize dangerous or unhealthy situations and interactions, which leads us to enter or stay in relationships that are chaotic and harmful because they seem familiar and safe. We may veer, with little warning, from a state of little feeling into a state of heightened feeling. We may give too much in a relationship or to needy friends or family, because we're emotionally unattuned to our own interior cues that should tell us we need to draw stronger boundaries—then we may erupt in anger when we realize that we're giving more than we're receiving.

―

Lanius helps patients who have experienced trauma in their youth to be aware of their feelings again—often for the first time (we'll read more about that in Chapter Seven). "Many of them have never felt positive emotions—they have a complete inability to experience positive feelings, and when they do feel something positive, they're immediately flooded with negative emotions," she says.

This is borne out by a study that found that kids who lost a parent early in life didn't necessarily have more negative moods than other people did—they simply had fewer *positive* moods. Investigators showed study participants forty mood words. People who lost a parent early in life experienced the negative words as negative, but, according to brainwave measurements, they also experienced the positive words they saw ("loving, warm-hearted, affectionate, pleased, happy, enthusiastic") as negative. Other research shows that kids who lost a parent at an early age later experience low self-esteem, loneliness, isolation, and an inability to express feelings—even seventy-one years after losing their parent.

Brain scans show that individuals who lack emotional awareness have lost interconnected neurocircuitry in critical areas. The more emotionally unaware these individuals are, the less activation they show not only in the default mode network but also in an area of the brain known as the "insula," a region involved in introceptive awareness—how aware we are of our bodily cues that tune us into what's happening to us at the moment. For example, we might be walking down a dark street and suddenly have a heightened sense that something is wrong because of our physical sensations: the hair on our arms is pricking up, our heartbeat becomes rapid. We realize we're feeling panicky—even before we hear the footsteps behind us. The body sends us these signals to tell us we could be in danger so that we'll react to protect ourselves.

Lanius has also found that those who have a dampened sense of emotionality show less activity in an area of the cortex, which indicates that "they are not self-reflective; they are not aware of what they feel emotionally, nor are they able to reflect on it mindfully."

This lack of awareness of feelings, this lack of consciousness as to how you might be contributing to disharmony or friction in a relationship, presents a problem for partners and parents, since the only way to manage your own stuff is to first be aware of what your stuff is. Without awareness, you can't be conscious of your behavior, and without being conscious of your behavior, you really don't know how to improve your interactions in your most meaningful life relationships.

Lanius's fMRI studies also show that early trauma decreases activity in an area of the brain that affects our ability to regulate and modulate emotions. When we have difficulty regulating our emotions and rebounding from stress, we are more easily "kindled" into anger. We may overreact to what we perceive as rejection, or injustice, or have a knee-jerk reaction to disagreements and discord. We may become hyper-aggressive, argumentative, defensive, and angry. When our emotions are underregulated, explains Lanius, "This decreased ability to dampen down intense feelings leads to greater activity in the amygdala, which regulates our emotional reactivity. Intense feeling states—anxiety, guilt, fear, shame, pain—increase." We react, big-time, to whoever or whatever is in front of us.

Or, we might react in the opposite way: feeling so hyperanxious and unable to process our feelings that we get quiet, we double down, passively retreating and avoiding confrontation at all costs. We may feel overwhelmed by feelings of loss and betrayal.

Most often, people with a history of early adversity go in between two mind states: overmodulation of feelings, shutting down emotionally because they're unaware of what they're truly feeling; and undermodulation, where they're caught up in intense feeling states and intense emotions, easily triggered by difficult interactions.

Those who've had multiple traumas in childhood might have multiple areas of thwarted brain development that affect them in myriad ways in adult life. They may be entirely clueless about their own behavior and how it affects others. "Given that they may have poor emotional awareness in general, they may not even know that they're caught going back and forth between these two mind states," says Lanius.

Attachment to Others Is a Biological Process

Attachment occurs when infants or young children are hungry, or wet, or afraid and learn that someone cares for them and will attend to their needs. They are safe.

In most cases, when an infant's or child's needs are met—he is fed, his diaper is changed, his parent soothes him—he develops secure attachment, little by little, event after event. When he is regularly soothed after feeling needy or afraid, he eventually learns how to calm himself down.

The brain circuits that regulate human behavior, and give a child a sense of who he is, and that he matters—so that he forms a sense of self and a connection with other people—develop as caregivers respond to that child's needs. These early relationships activate the growth of all the various regions of our brain that we need to use in order to have healthy relationships.

A baby smiles, a mom coos, a baby coos back, the mom smiles. In this one small moment, the mother attunes to and reflects back what her infant is expressing. And this experience—being seen and known—becomes encoded in the infant's neural circuitry.

But if a child's basic needs for safety and security aren't met, she will reach adulthood without ever having learned what it means to be soothed in healthy ways—or how to calm herself down—when she meets inevitable life and relationship stressors. She will have an insecure sense of attachment.

Most psychologists agree that a child has to develop a secure attachment with at least one primary caregiver in order to learn how to effectively regulate her own emotions for the rest of her life, and in order to learn how to become attached in a healthy way in adult relationships.

Most people with attachment issues can't understand why others are reluctant to get as close to them as they'd like; they instead feel this synaptic disconnect in the form of rejection and isolation. Think of Kat. "No relationship ever stuck for me in my twenties and early thirties, and I always thought it was the other person's problem. It's only now, looking back, that I realize I had this huge reactivity, and can take responsibility for how I behaved." Kat can see now that she'd often be anxious, "a bottomless pit of need" for reassurance, then become "sarcastic or passive-aggressive if my partner wasn't giving me enough emotional stroking." At the same time, if someone got too close to Kat, she couldn't sustain it. "Something small would happen in a relationship and all the sadness and fear and panic I'd felt when I was young would just come spilling out. Before I knew it, I'd be critical, blaming, controlling, and in-your-face argumentative." Each time a relationship "imploded badly," it reinforced Kat's conclusions that others didn't—and couldn't—love her.

And so the underconnected areas of Kat's brain stayed offline for a very long time.

As for John, psychologists would see his profound need for closeness, and his sabotaging of it, as a sign of his early insecure attachment with his dad.

A history of insecure attachment also affects what kind of parents we become. Recently, researchers at the University of Minnesota's Institute of Child Development followed seventy-three children from birth into young adulthood.

Kids whose parents had not soothed them effectively behaved quite differently in their grown-up romantic relationships from kids who'd had warmer, more supportive parents. Young adults who'd been less attached to their parents when small had more trouble managing their negative, reactive feelings and recovering from conflict with their adult partners. Children who had had secure attachments with loving, even-keeled parents were far better at recovering from adult conflict. They were able to manage their fear or anger before those feelings overwhelmed them—and then move on.

Not surprisingly, these kids who'd had secure attachments with their mothers also had healthier love relationships and reported being a lot happier in them over the long term.

In a similar longitudinal study, researchers followed Oregon families for three generations. Parents who were warm, consistent, not overreactive, and involved in their kids' activities had a positive impact not only on how their adolescent children turned out but also on how skilled their kids were, once grown, in using positive parenting skills with their own children. Positive parenting habits, and being able to manage one's reactivity in family life, transferred to the next generation of children and even grandchildren.

In another large study, nearly a thousand men and women between the ages of twenty-five and seventy-four said their childhood relationships with their mothers had been better than their relationships with their fathers—and this was especially true for boys. We don't know why this is—perhaps there is some truth to the saying that dads are harder on their sons. But men who had enjoyed a good relationship with their dads during childhood were less emotionally reactive to stressful events in their daily lives as adults than were men who'd had poor relationships with their fathers. Other studies have found that sons who have fond childhood memories of their dads are more able to stay emotionally calm and stable in the face of everyday stressors.

In a twenty-five-year study, researchers followed boys from the age of nine until they were thirty-three years old. By then, many had started their own families. Those men whose dads had poor parenting methods were, predictably, less skilled parents themselves. Boys whose dads' behavior had been categorized as hostile; angry; threatening; neglectful, as in not knowing where their son was and not taking an active role in his life and activities; or lacking consistent follow-through behaved very differently with everyone around them. They were less able to create healthy, caring bonds and relationships with teachers and peers, coaches and mentors. They had fewer positive connections with *anyone*, and were more likely to be seen as antisocial and to connect with other teens who were negative influences upon them.

Later, when these boys had their own families, they were inconsistent and ineffective parents and their own children displayed more negative and challenging behaviors than did other kids.

Poor parenting leads to insecurity and less-healthy love relationships in adulthood. Constructive parenting over generations passes on good parenting skills and gives kids a foundation for seeking out other positive influences and mentors; kids relate better with others and create good relationships that help them to be happy, well adjusted, and successful. And, later, they and their healthy partners raise good enough families.

Stories like John's make sense. But what's entirely new in our understanding of how family dysfunction is inherited is the discovery that poor parenting styles—which foster childhood adversity—also engender biological changes in children's brains that make those kids neurobiologically less able to be good partners and parents when they reach adulthood.

Family dysfunction and familial loss become a neurobiological inheritance.

It's a generational feedback loop: if our parents were highly reactive, we're more likely to be a reactive partner, or marry a reactive partner, or be parents who are not evenhanded, raising kids who will bear their own scars and be reactive in their future family life.

We see this human truth borne out in popular movies and novels and plays. Donna Tartt's *The Goldfinch*, Tracy Letts's *August: Osage County*, all of Ibsen's and Chekhov's works, among many others, show that damaging relationships in childhood lead to damaging relationships in adulthood. We recognize the fact that childhood Chronic Unpredictable Toxic Stress can change us, which makes these fictional characters' stories and fates so compelling.

———

When we grow up without secure attachment, we will not be wired for love. As attachment researcher Louis Cozolino writes, we are not the survival of the fittest; we are the survival of the nurtured, and "those who are nurtured best survive best."

It makes sense that people who repeatedly make poor decisions in choosing partners and have troubled relationships keep repeating their mistakes. Their motivations are as biological as they are emotional. The woman who can't stop blaming her husband for every small infraction, the man who can't stop trying to control his wife: their brains didn't receive the love needed to foster the critical neural interconnections that create secure, loving attachment. They keep bumping up against the same neurobiological deficits, over and over again.

But that's not the entire story. It turns out, happily, that we can repair and regrow the underdeveloped neurobiological connections that were long ago interrupted in childhood—so that we can at last enjoy the kinds of relationships, and family life, we long for.

PART II

Recovering from Post Childhood
Adversity Syndrome: How Do We
Come Back to Who We Really Are?

CHAPTER SIX

Beginning Your Healing Journey

Recognizing that chronic childhood stress leads to chronic adult illness and relationship challenges can be enormously freeing. If you have been wondering why you've been struggling a little too hard for a little too long with your emotional and physical well-being—feeling as if you've been swimming against some invisible current that never ceases—this aha can come as a welcome relief. Finally, you can *see* the current. And you see how it's been working steadily against you all of your life.

At last you understand how the past spills into the present and a tough childhood can become a tumultuous, challenging adulthood. As Laura—whom we met in the first chapter of this book—put it so well when she learned about Adverse Childhood Experiences for the first time, "Now I understand why I've felt all my life as if I've been trying to dance without hearing any music."

There is truth to the old saying that knowledge is power. Once you understand that your body and brain have been deeply affected, you can at last take the necessary, science-based steps to remove the fingerprints that early adversity has left on your neurobiology. You can reduce your proclivity to inflammation, depression, addiction, physical pain, and disease.

You have a choice either to stay locked in the past, thinking of what might have been, or to proactively help yourself and those you love, embrace resilience and move forward toward growth, even transformation.

———

Editors of the mental health diagnostic bible known as the *DSM-V* (*Diagnostic and Statistical Manual of Mental Disorders*, 5th edition) recently considered including a new diagnosis, "Developmental Trauma Disorder." This term recognizes the long-lasting impact that chronic, unpredictable Adverse Childhood Experiences has on later mental and physical health and well-being.

Because understanding of the diagnostic signs and possible treatments for Developmental Trauma Disorder is still evolving, it was not included in the *DSM*. Yet, even Developmental Trauma Disorder doesn't fully speak to the deep, invisible, and subtle ways in which we now know that childhood Chronic Unpredictable Toxic Stressors change us on a biological level and lead to chronic illness.

I propose calling this challenge Post Childhood Adversity Syndrome. We don't really need a diagnostic label to grasp how the long arm of childhood suffering extends from the past to grip us in the present. Yet the name might prove helpful as we examine strategies for healing.

In the following three chapters, we're going to look at what today's top experts tell us about how to undo the impact of Post Childhood Adversity Syndrome.

———

Science tells us that biology does not have to be destiny. ACEs can last a lifetime but they don't have to. We can reboot our brains. Just as physical wounds and bruises heal, just as we can regain our muscle tone, we can recover function in underconnected areas of the brain. The brain and body are never static; they are always in the process of becoming and changing.

Even if we have been set on high reactive mode for decades or a lifetime, we can still dial it down. We can respond to life's inevitable stressors more appropriately and shift away from an overactive inflammatory response. We can become neurobiologically resilient. We can turn bad epigenetics into good epigenetics and rescue ourselves.

Today, scientists recognize a range of promising approaches to help create new neurons (known as neurogenesis), make new synaptic connections between those neurons (known as synaptogenesis), promote new patterns of thoughts and reactions, bring underconnected areas of the brain back online—and reset our stress response so that we decrease the inflammation that makes us ill.

We have the capacity, within ourselves, to create better health. We might call this brave undertaking "the neurobiology of awakening."

In this chapter, we'll examine steps you can take on your own, right now, to jump-start healing. Some you can do in your own living room; others require taking a course or utilizing online resources. In Chapter Seven, we'll look at approaches that require professional support, and in Chapter Eight, we'll examine parenting strategies.

A Healing Journey: Twelve Steps to Help You Come Back to Who You Really Are

1. Take the ACE Survey

A critical first step before setting out on a healing journey is to take the Adverse Childhood Experiences Survey, and calculate your ACE Score. You can find the survey on page xxi or online at www.acestudy .org/survey.

One of the authors of the ACE Study, Dr. Vincent Felitti, hopes that making the survey available to everyone online will help to dispel any secrecy and shame associated with ACEs. For many people, he says, answering the questionnaire "helps to normalize the conversation about Adverse Childhood Experiences and their impact on our lives. When we make it okay to talk about what happened, it removes the power that secrecy so often has."

After taking the survey, and computing your ACE Score, ask yourself the following questions:

How old was I at the time of these events? The earlier that certain patterns of adversity began, the more difficult it is for a child to understand his or her situation or find help.

Is it likely that there are events I don't remember? Many Adverse Childhood Experiences happen before we are old enough to store those memories. Some of your responses may be based more on your implicit memory—how you feel—rather than your explicit memory, or your recall of specific events. No one can remember what happened in the first years of life. You may have implicit memories that are "known but not remembered." Yet they still wield an influence over you that are just as powerful as explicit memories. You may not remember them but you still relive them. Think of situations that make you uncomfortable and see if you can track back to a reason for your unease.

What was my relationship to the person or persons involved in the adversity I faced? Was someone you trusted and depended on for your survival a source of chronic, unpredictable stress?

How much support did I receive from other caregivers in my life? If, for instance, one parent was unreliable, was there another parent or family member who looked out for you, to whom you were emotionally attached?

As you consider the answers to these questions, think about sharing your findings with a person you trust, to see if he or she has further insights. You might also consider taking your completed survey—either in this book or printed out if you did it online—into your next exam with your physician or health-care practitioner. Explain to him or her that you believe there may be a direct association between the chronic, unpredictable stress you faced when you were young and the chronic conditions you face today. Ask for your physician's thoughts.

Felitti believes that if enough patients do this, we will increase societal awareness of the impact that Adverse Childhood Experiences have on adult well-being and start to change medicine from "the patient up."

Let's be clear: you're not asking your health-care practitioner to step in as a therapist (we'll get to therapy later) or to change prescriptions or suggestions for your care. The goal is simply to let him know of the link between your past and your present. Ideally, your health-care practitioner will acknowledge, given so much recent scientific research in this field, that such a link is entirely plausible, and add some of the modalities we're about to explore to your healing protocol.

Felitti tells his patients who have suffered ACEs, "I understand. I acknowledge their story and that it happened—and that it's connected to what is happening to them right now." To have what has for so long gone unsaid spoken and affirmed aloud can, in and of itself, provide patients with a sense of instantaneous relief. That awareness of your experience, and acceptance of you as a person, can mark the beginning of a change. In that moment, Felitti says, "A mechanism, and momentum, for healing is set in place, even for seemingly intractable chronic conditions. Just one conversation about the fact that ACEs matter in a patient's current health can have enormously beneficial output. *Asking*, including about subjects we have been taught as children that nice people don't discuss, *Listening*, and *Accepting* that patient for who they are, in all their human complexity, are a powerful form of *Doing* that confers great relief to patients."

Felitti has seen, over and over again, that, "Once a patient is able to say that something happened to them when they were small, they begin to heal."

2. Find Out Your Resilience Score

The resilience survey below is based on resilience research and was developed by a group of researchers, therapists, pediatricians, and physicians. It is available online at http://ACEsTooHigh.com.

RESILIENCE QUESTIONNAIRE

Please circle the most accurate answer under each statement:

1. I believe that my mother loved me when I was little.

| Definitely true | Probably true | Not sure | Probably not true | Definitely not true |

2. I believe that my father loved me when I was little.

| Definitely true | Probably true | Not sure | Probably not true | Definitely not true |

3. When I was little, other people helped my mother and father take care of me and they seemed to love me.

| Definitely true | Probably true | Not sure | Probably not true | Definitely not true |

4. I've heard that when I was an infant someone in my family enjoyed playing with me, and I enjoyed it, too.

| Definitely true | Probably true | Not sure | Probably not true | Definitely not true |

5. When I was a child, there were relatives in my family who made me feel better if I was sad or worried.

Definitely true	Probably true	Not sure	Probably not true	Definitely not true

6. When I was a child, neighbors or my friends' parents seemed to like me.

Definitely true	Probably true	Not sure	Probably not true	Definitely not true

7. When I was a child, teachers, coaches, youth leaders, or ministers were there to help me.

Definitely true	Probably true	Not sure	Probably not true	Definitely not true

8. Someone in my family cared about how I was doing in school.

Definitely true	Probably true	Not sure	Probably not true	Definitely not true

9. My family, neighbors, and friends talked often about making our lives better.

Definitely true	Probably true	Not sure	Probably not true	Definitely not true

10. We had rules in our house and were expected to keep them.

Definitely true	Probably true	Not sure	Probably not true	Definitely not true

11. When I felt really bad, I could almost always find someone I trusted to talk to.

Definitely true	Probably true	Not sure	Probably not true	Definitely not true

12. When I was a youth, people noticed that I was capable and could get things done.

Definitely true	Probably true	Not sure	Probably not true	Definitely not true

13. I was independent and a go-getter.

Definitely true	Probably true	Not sure	Probably not true	Definitely not true

14. I believed that life is what you make it.

Definitely true	Probably true	Not sure	Probably not true	Definitely not true

How many of these fourteen protective factors did I have as a child and youth? (How many of the fourteen were circled "Definitely True" or "Probably True"?)

_____

Of these circled, how many are still true for me? _____

As with the ACE Survey, the Resilience Survey gives insight into your personal story—in this case highlighting what your strengths are. As you set out to speak your truth, the positive aspects of your childhood experiences are an essential part of your story.

According to Jane Stevens, journalist and founder of the social network ACEsConnection.com and the news site ACEsTooHigh.com, "It's important for people to calculate their resilience score as well as their ACE Score so that they can understand what helped them withstand adversity in their childhood, and consider how they might incorporate more resilience factors in their adult lives."

3. Write to Heal

Even if you have no health-care practitioner to share your story with, you can begin to speak your truth by "writing to heal." This creates the experience of seeing yourself for who you really are, perhaps for the first time in your life.

Bernie Siegel, MD, often uses the "writing to heal" exercise in workshops. Recently, he asked a group of high schoolers to write letters to themselves on the topic of "why you love yourself." Then he had them write letters to themselves on a more bracing topic: why they might want to end their lives. Siegel wanted students to see, at the end of his experiment, that the pile of pages the entire group of teens had written on why they thought they should commit suicide was five times higher than the pile on why they thought they should love themselves.

"It was only at that point, once they knew they were not alone with their painful emotions, that they were able to not lie about what it was that they felt, and start creating lives for themselves," says Siegel. He learned in his thirty years as an assistant clinical professor of general and pediatric surgery at Yale, that "whether your story is about having met with emotional pain or physical pain, the important thing is to take the lid off of those feelings. When you keep your emotions repressed, that's when the body starts to try to get your attention. Because *you* aren't paying attention. Our childhood is stored up in our bodies, and one day, the body will present its bill."

Felitti often asks patients, "Before you come back for your next appointment, start sending me a detailed history of your life."

Studies show that writing about stressful experiences not only helps patients to get better, it keeps them from getting worse. James Pennebaker, PhD, psychology professor at the University of Texas at Austin, developed this simple assignment: "Over the next four days, write down your deepest emotions and thoughts about the emotional upheaval that has been influencing your life the most. In your writing, really let go and explore the event and how it has affected you. You might tie this experience to your childhood, your relationship with your parents, people you have loved or love now, or even your career. Write continuously for twenty minutes a day."

According to Pennebaker, even "short-term focused writing can have a beneficial effect." For instance, when students were asked to write to heal, their grades went up. When individuals wrote about emotional upheavals, they went to the doctor less and showed changes in immune function. The exercise of simply writing about your secrets, even if you destroy your writing immediately afterward, has been shown to have a positive effect on health, even for people battling life-threatening diseases.

Researchers at Carnegie Mellon found that the simple act of writing and reporting on an emotional state had a substantial impact on the body's physical state. They had participants complete a difficult math task while evaluators gave them negative criticism that was intended to make participants feel angry and ashamed. Afterward, one group wrote about their emotional state and the other didn't. Those who wrote about their anger and frustration for just a few minutes had a smaller increase in heart rate, and a healthier cardiovascular response, than those who didn't express themselves.

—

Kendall, who suffered from undiagnosed celiac disease and was teased and belittled by her family, decided to write a document outlining the reality and facts of her health situation as a child, along with her parents' "damaging response." She wrote the letter because her parents were asking to have more contact with her family, which she wasn't comfortable with.

Kendall gave the document to her therapist, who then met with Kendall's parents to discuss it with them. "I do not have the health, energy, or inclination to reestablish a relationship with my parents at this point," Kendall says. "But I did need to write up the document for my well-being, as well as to give my parents some needed information." Since writing the document, two things have changed in Kendall's health situation. "For the first time since my diagnosis, my celiac disease is no longer considered refractory," she says. "Results from my recent upper GI endoscopy show that my villi have healed."

Kat also decided to write down her story. "It was hard for me because we were always shunned in my family whenever we mentioned what had happened. But I suddenly realized I needed to give myself permission to tell my truth," she says. "I wanted to rewrite my story and tell it from my perspective in order to give my story meaning." So Kat began. "Here I was, pushing thirty-five, broke and broken, drowning in a deluge of memories. I was still carrying around that feeling from that first moment when I saw my mother's body, that terror and grief. I had never let it all surface, and I was unable to let it all go."

She wrote down every memory, every emotion, as well as her experiences as she set out to heal herself. She self-published the book *I Think I'll Make It: A True Story of Lost and Found* and shared it with all of her family members as well as the world. In writing, she was able to let go of her guilt and shame. "Writing was an enormously healing process," she says.

Today, Kat is a motivational speaker and life coach who gives talks to high school students about overcoming adversity—using her voice to tell a truth that, for so many decades, could never be told.

4. Draw It

You can also draw pictures in order to "bring forth the wounds," advises Bernie Siegel, MD. Draw anything that comes to mind. Says Siegel, "You might choose to draw an outdoor scene, or a picture of your family. See what images come up. Then put your drawing away and look at it the next day to analyze it; think of it as if you were interpreting a dream. Does it give you any insights?"

Siegel recalls a patient who drew an attractive female figure in great detail and also drew, in the background, a small clock, of seemingly little consequence, on the wall. The clock had only one hand, which pointed to the number 12. "Her unconscious was demanding that she pay attention to a past childhood experience that was traumatic, one that had happened when she was twelve," Siegel says.

Another woman Siegel treated had severe pelvic pain. She had seen many doctors, none of whom could find a medical cause for her pain. So Siegel asked her to draw a picture. She drew a heart that looked like a valentine, cracked down the middle, dripping blood. Siegel counted the drops of blood—there were twenty-one. "And so I asked her, what happened when you were twenty-one years old?" She revealed the story of her trauma, and began to find relief for her physical pain.

We don't entirely understand the science of how "art therapy" can unmask past trauma, but psychologists sometimes find it a useful tool to uncover what the subconscious mind has hidden away.

In Chapter Seven, we'll look at healing steps we can take with the help of professionals. Save any drawings or writing you're moved to do in case you seek outside support; these may prove helpful to your healing process.

5. Mindfulness Meditation—the Best Method for Repairing the Brain

Brain scans of individuals who faced childhood adversity often show a loss of interconnectivity in areas that are critical to creating loving relationships, activating a sense of calm in the face of stress, and downshifting the inflammatory response. When these connections are underdeveloped, we have little awareness of our own feelings and lack consciousness about the effects of our behavior on others. We can't see how our defensive patterns of interacting are hurting those we care for—and we can't see how they are hurting us. We lack insight into how to improve our relationships. We are limited. Our happiness is limited. We limit the happiness of others.

Mindfulness meditation helps to change our brain—and to bring the brain back online and reset our inflammation response. In one recent study, individuals who practiced mindfulness meditation and mindfulness-based stress reduction (MBSR) during a one-day, eight-hour retreat demonstrated physical changes that reduced their response to stress and their levels of inflammatory hormones. They were able to recover faster from stress and they were less reactive to stress. They still pumped out inflammatory hormones such as cortisol when stressed, but their cortisol levels went down more quickly once the stressor had passed. Faster "cortisol recovery" means you can rebound more quickly from stressful situations. It means that you reduce the time that your body and mind are bathed in inflammatory chemicals. This leads to less physical and neural inflammation and less physical disease, anxiety, and depression. Meditation can help you learn to calm your mind, and increase emotional and physical well-being even if you came of age amid a range of Adverse Childhood Experiences.

Dr. Ryan Herringa, assistant professor of child and adolescent psychiatry at the University of Wisconsin, says that this is true for kids, too. "When kids practice mindfulness they may strengthen the same circuits of the brain weakened by early adversity and childhood trauma—including the frontal lobe and the hippocampus."

Mindfulness meditation has been shown to help individuals regulate emotions, respond flexibly to others, evaluate options, and make appropriate decisions. It also increases empathy, self-awareness, and self-reflection, and helps relieve feelings of fearfulness. When you become aware of your breath and bodily sensations, you trigger an underlying mechanism that helps you to regulate and reduce painful feelings.

According to Trish Magyari, LCPC, a mindfulness-based psychotherapist and researcher who specializes in trauma and illness, adults suffering from PTSD due to childhood sexual abuse who took part in a "trauma-sensitive" mindfulness-based stress reduction (MBSR) program, showed less anxiety, depression, and PTSD symptoms, and these improvements lasted even two years after taking the course. In another study, people who took an eight-week MBSR course showed an increase in the density and concentration of the gray matter of the hippocampus, the area associated with memory, processing emotions, and managing stress. MBSR training (which includes twenty-six hours of class time—usually eight short sessions and one all-day class) has also been shown to increase gray matter in the brain stem, helping to modulate the release of stress hormones.

In other words, meditation may help repopulate the brain with gray matter—and the neurons that may have been pruned so many years ago.

These are stunning health benefits from a very simple practice: you focus on your breath, note and name your thoughts, let them go, and see that you are not your thoughts. You free yourself from worrying, spinning stories, and ruminating, in order to be in the present moment. You free yourself from your inflammatory responses.

When you breathe deeply and bring oxygen into your lungs, that oxygen travels throughout the body, into the cells, where it supports all life-giving biological pathways. As you breathe in and out with long, slow breaths through mindful breathing, you also strengthen and recharge the activity of your underactive parasympathetic nervous system. Although physicians can prescribe many medications that can dampen the activity of the sympathetic nervous system, including valium and SSRIs, there is no medication that can help to boost the parasympathetic nervous system. Your breath is the best calming treatment known.

To establish a daily meditation practice, it's important to start with an attitude of unconditional friendliness toward yourself, and give permission for the meditation experience to be whatever it is, says Tara Brach, PhD, meditation teacher and psychologist.

Set a regular time and space for your daily sitting. You can sit on a chair or a cushion on the floor, whatever is most comfortable. Be aware of your posture, so that you can remain alert and awake. Allow your hands to rest comfortably on your knees or lap. "Close your eyes, relax, and let go," says Brach. Take several full deep breaths, and with each exhalation, consciously let go, relaxing the face, shoulders, hands, and belly area. Consciously releasing body tension will help you open to whatever arises during your meditation. "You might take a few minutes at the beginning of your meditation to scan through the body with your attention, softening and becoming aware of sensations from the inside out," she suggests. Listen to sounds with your senses open. Feel the space around you in and outside the room.

Choose a primary anchor for your meditation: you might choose to focus on the breath as it enters and leaves the nostrils; the rise and fall of your chest; sensations in your hands or through the whole body; or sounds within or around you.

When you notice that you have drifted off and become lost in thought, come back to your anchor. You might, Brach suggests, "Rest in the inflow and outflow of the breath as your home base, and also be mindful of the sounds in the room, a feeling of sleepiness, an itch, heat."

Dan Siegel, MD, offers this helpful image. Imagine your awareness as a great wheel. At the hub of the wheel is your mindful sense of awareness, and from this hub, many spokes extend out to the rim. You've been conditioned to move your attention away from that sense of inner awareness, out along the spokes, and to affix it to one part of the rim after another. You judge yourself for what you said in a phone conversation a few hours earlier; you remember a scene with your mother from when you were ten; your neck hurts; you feel trepidation over an upcoming doctor's appointment, anger at your spouse for not helping with dinner. You get caught up in spinning stories about what you or others did wrong. If you are not connected to your hub, your sense of inner awareness, if your attention is trapped out on the rim, you are cut off from yourself, living in what Tara Brach calls "a trance."

Training in mindfulness allows you to return to the still center of the wheel and live your moments with full awareness.

As you begin to practice meditation, remember that getting distracted is natural. When a thought arises, notice it and name it: here is worrying, here is judging. Then let it go.

"Just as the body secretes enzymes, the mind generates thoughts," Brach explains. Thoughts are not the enemy. "When you recognize that you have been lost in thought, relax back into the actual experience of being Here. Listen to sounds, re-relax your shoulders, hands, and belly, and relax your heart. Arrive again in mindful presence, senses wide open. Notice the difference between any thought and the vividness of this Here-ness."

For Kat, one of her most profound turning points in healing came from mindfulness meditation. "I'd watched a movie called *Dharma Brothers*, about how *vipassana* meditation was helping individuals in the Alabama State prison to forgive themselves. Inmates said that learning meditation was the most rewarding, healing, and empowering thing they had ever done. They realized that they were not the sum of what had happened to them in life. And I thought, if it can help them to find peace after so much violence, maybe it can help me."

Kat read books on emotional healing by mindfulness meditation and Buddhist teachers, and realized that she was not the only one suffering; these wise teachers told stories of all kinds of trauma, and showed that the way out of that suffering was to embark on an inner path of self-awareness. Kat understood for the first time that she was not alone. Other people had felt the self-loathing, loss, and shame that she felt. "They may not have had my experiences, but they had suffered as I had suffered." Kat began to feel "deep down, that maybe I deserved healing, too. I began to experience this inexplicable, innate desire to come alive."

She realized, too, that "All this suffering had surfaced and I'd never stopped to examine that my body was holding on to my victimhood so tightly—as if for dear life. I had so much proof, based on my childhood experiences—that life hadn't been fair to me. I felt that I had every right to assume I'd never get to have the life I deserved, that bad stuff would always happen to me. I had a master's degree and I was valeting cars and bartending." She felt this was the limited life that someone like her would have, until she realized that she "*could* make the choice to go on a quest for healing."

Kat started practicing with a guided meditation tape for five minutes at a time, three times a day. Then she worked her way up to twice a day for twenty minutes. Over time, in the course of her practice, of getting very still, focusing on her breath, naming her thoughts, and letting them go, Kat had a set of life-changing experiences.

"I was sitting cross-legged on my bed. There was a huge thunderstorm. As I quieted my mind, the sound of the thunder brought back these deep, forgotten memories of childhood trips with my mom to a beach house on the Delaware shore when I was very small. I found myself rocking back and forth."

Kat couldn't understand why she was swaying as she meditated, so she asked herself, "Why am I rocking?" And the answer came to her: "I had this sense of my mom's presence, holding me. I just felt her there with me. And I began to experience this overwhelming gratitude to her—even though she hadn't been in my life for a long time—for being my mom, for loving me as she had. Then I began to feel my grandmother with me. And I felt this overwhelming gratitude for how she had loved me, protected me, during the years I lived with her. I felt a penetrating, warm glow permeate my skin, like a deep, chemical reaction was taking place throughout my body. I felt a sense of security and safety that I could not, at least in my conscious memory, ever remember having had before. Of being loved, really loved."

That feeling, Kat says, "opened me up to this wider sense that I was connected to something bigger than even the women who had loved me. I felt connected to a greater life presence, a kind of loving awareness. And suddenly that vacant feeling that had hollowed me out all my life, that grief that I was life's victim, abandoned, alone—it just lifted."

When Kat meditates, she says, "I feel a letting go of my personal history, like a weight lifting off of my body."

At one point, Kat went to a ten-day silent *vipassana* retreat in Virginia. "On the fifth day, we were doing a body scan, bringing our awareness to different areas in our body. I had been sitting so long that I was in utter pain. We were asked to focus our attention on our right eye. And tears just started to flow out of my right eye, only my right eye. And then we got to our neck," Kat says.

Kat's neck was not an area she wanted to focus on. "I have a thing about my neck," she explains. (Her father killed her mother by strangling her with his bare hands.) "I have somatized that memory," Kat says. "I have never liked anything that fits tight around my neck— clothing, jewelry. But here we were, focusing on the neck, breathing. I began to feel my body welling up. All the pain in my body just began to grow larger and larger. It was as if I had embodied everything that had happened and all this negative energy had been stored in the cells of my body. Bringing my focus to my neck triggered pain I'd hidden for so long."

After that meditation session, Kat began sobbing uncontrollably. "I could not stop the flood of raw emotion. It was excruciating, but it also felt good. I was ready to be cleansed." She could barely get up off the floor. "I struggled to my feet. I was like Bambi, I couldn't walk, and I was still sobbing as I made it to the door of the meditation hall. I looked outside and saw a tree. And it was suddenly as if I'd never seen a tree before," she says. "Everything was new."

That's when Kat realized that "I had let go of my pain, my story of loss, my victimhood, the grief and fear and sense of failure and shame and guilt from so much abandonment. I had to say good-bye to all the negative emotions that I had embodied over the years. Because when I let go, I was greeted by a new, deeper layer of wholeness, a sense of inner freedom.

"I began to notice things I hadn't noticed before: things as simple as the beauty of the sun shining, or moments when I was with someone and we were laughing. I began to connect with the world around me as if I were seeing the beauty in the world for the first time. I began to wake up."

As Kat began to see things around her more clearly, she learned to put a pause between her feelings and her actions. She gained a sense of what her triggers were, of what was going on deep inside her, her patterns, and the ways in which she was working against herself. This led to her ability to have her first healthy love relationship.

Today, Kat is engaged to a woman with whom she has an honest and deeply loving relationship.

"I think I rewrote the story of my brain," Kat says. "And that allowed me to rewrite the story of how I loved."

Other individuals whose stories appear in these pages likewise found solace in meditation and mindfulness. Ellie, who grew up navigating a violent world in which her much older brothers were often incarcerated, came to mindfulness and meditation practice as a way to "clearly see how my current thoughts about my lack of self-worth are connected to my long-ago past, so that I could try to get my intrusive, everyday thoughts of how worthless I am to budge—to move out." It has been very powerful for her to pay attention to "not only what I am thinking but how I am responding to my thoughts."

Mindfulness has been "life changing" for Ellie. "I have been to many therapists who've helped me to analyze my feelings, but no one had ever said that it was possible to simply let my thoughts pass, so that I could experience the freedom of seeing that I am not my thoughts."

Meditation allows you to come to terms with your past so that you can live in the present, be here, and enjoy what is right here, right now.

—

A daily ten-minute practice of mindfulness meditation can be an act of mental hygiene that dramatically down-regulates your stress response.

The best place to start is to look for a local class on either mindfulness-based stress reduction (MBSR) or an Insight Meditation Group, taught by a skilled teacher. Luckily, many community centers, yoga studios, and hospitals now offer MBSR and insight meditation classes for affordable fees. Some offer MBSR discounts and scholarships for those in special circumstances, and most libraries have a wide range of meditation CDs available.

To find an MBSR class near you, visit the Center for Mindfulness in Medicine, Health Care and Society—found on the University of Massachusetts Medical School website at www.umassmed.edu/MBSR/public/searchmember.aspx. MBSR was designed initially to assist people with pain and life issues that were difficult to treat in a hospital setting, and utilizes a combination of mindfulness meditation, mindful awareness, mindful movement, and yoga.

The Insight Meditation Society offers instructions and guidance in insight meditation, also known as *vipassana*, a form of meditation that is in the Buddhist tradition. The simple technique focuses attention on the breath, helping to calm the mind so that you can more clearly see your own thought patterns, become aware of your mental conditioning and how it may be working against you, and learn to be more fully present in the moment. You can learn more about a wide array of workshops, community meditation programs, and retreats with some of the world's most renowned meditation teachers at www.dharma.org/.

Hundreds of terrific *vipassana* insight meditations and downloadable podcasts are also available free (or for a donation) online. I've been most helped by the work of Tara Brach, PhD; Sylvia Boorstein, PhD; Jack Kornfield, PhD; Sharon Salzberg; Trish Magyari (who teaches MBSR); Norman Fischer; and Pema Chödrön; their guided meditations and teachings have been life-changing for me.

6. Tai Chi and Qigong

In his search for healing, John gravitated toward tai chi and qigong, also known as moving meditation. He began with a class at a tai chi school near his house, and quickly found that when he practiced the slow, measured movements of tai chi, he felt a new sense of calm come over him. When he began his practice, he found that he "would go in very wound up, but after forty-five minutes of slow, careful movement, my inner ruminating voice would fall silent. I'd put all of my focus on what I was doing. And little by little, I began to create a space to recuperate, to find clarity of mind, to see things more clearly—in my relationships, in my work, and in my thoughts about myself. And that clarity became a powerful tool to help me manage my stress reactions, my fears and insecurities. Instead of taking a defensive stance, or blaming others, I maintain perspective. I have become more compassionate. I see that the past was past. I have been able to see that the only thing that has been holding me back from healing, and achieving what I want to achieve, has been me. That voice that I've been hearing so long—my father's voice telling me, 'You're not good enough'—that voice is only a voice in my head."

In the two years that John has been practicing moving meditation, he says, "I have made so much progress in my health. I am in a different place. The chronic fatigue is gone. I have energy again. I'm running and hiking again. I recently ran several 5 and 10Ks. I can eat food again. I feel like I have come back."

Recently, John began spending more time with his dad—even taking him to a tai chi class with him. The results of these efforts to communicate with the man who caused most of John's childhood adversity have been surprising. "When I am with my dad now, and he gets worked up about something small, I don't react. I don't lose it. And I can see that my dad has learned how to step back, and calm himself down, and even apologize. I've been able to see that the man my dad was, this person I have been so angry with and in fear of and reacting to in my mind all these years, my dad is just not 'that guy' anymore. I have changed, and he has been quietly changing, too."

John, his parents, and his younger brother have started taking family vacations together. "We have decided, as a family, that we aren't interested in giving each other gifts for holidays and birthdays." Instead, John says, "We want to give each other new memories to replace our less happy ones," he says. "We have a really good time. We enjoy being together now."

This new relationship with his former tormentor has had a trickle-up, healing impact, helping John to both heal from his past and have hope for the future.

"We are the Good Enough Family," John says. And being part of a good enough family gives John hope that he may one day have a good enough family of his own.

7. Mindsight

"The brain is our enabler—our control center," says Dan Siegel, MD. He encourages those who've faced adversity to develop what he calls "Mindsight," the ability to truly see or know the mind. When you focus your attention on the mind and how it's working, it's possible to build specific circuits, repair neurocircuitry, and grow connections among neurons in the same areas of the brain that tend to be weak due to early adversity, trauma, and insecure attachment.

The first aspect of Mindsight is insight, the ability to sense your own inner mental life and reflect inwardly—what you might think of as being self-aware or self-knowing. The second is empathy, the ability to sense the inner mental life of another person—knowing who that person is. And the third is integration, the ability to link those two awarenesses and other processes into an interconnected big picture.

Integration helps you to approach problems reflectively and interact with others in healthy, wise ways. It promotes compassionate connections and communications. It helps you to reconnect your past, present, and future in a coherent way so that your life story makes sense of who you are. Siegel explains, "Mindsight enables us to go beyond 'being sad' or 'being angry' and to recognize that we have these feelings of sadness or anger, see that they are not the totality of who we are, accept them for what they are, and then allow them to transform so they do not lead to depression or anger and rage."

When you are aware of what you're feeling, when you are in tune with your inner world, you recognize when you're getting primed to react, you notice that your heart rate is going up, your breathing is shallow, your muscles are tense, so you pause. You take a deep breath, take a break; you let yourself calm down.

When you develop Mindsight, you make new neurons and new synaptic connections; increase your gray matter; and increase your myelin, making new white matter. "Tuning in to your own thoughts and those of others links different aspects of the brain and body that help with your capacity to be attuned to the world around you in a new way," says Siegel. "This allows for both personal well-being, and healthier relationships."

You don't need to go to a training camp to start this important process. You can simply start where you are by regularly reflecting on your inner life and being more reflective during conversations.

Try this exercise: Close your eyes and ask yourself, "What am I sensing right now in my body?" You may feel tension in your muscles or you may sense your heart beating, your lungs breathing. You may feel a wave of physical sensations. What images come up in your mind's eye? What feelings are inside you? You might try this the next time you're feeling stressed or are in a stressful conversation.

When you examine feelings and thoughts, these mental activities create energy in the brain. "Ions flowing in and out of the membranes of our brain's basic cells, our neurons, lead to the release of chemicals that allow these neurons to communicate with one another," Siegel says. That electrochemical energy helps to reconnect areas of the brain that are less connected due to early adversity, stimulating the growth of neurons and strengthening the brain.

"Families that have Mindsight are resilient," says Siegel.

If you begin to practice Step 5—meditation—you're already starting to create connections among neurons that integrate the brain. The next few steps are also great ways to help develop Mindsight.

8. Loving-kindness

Meditation changes your relationship to your thoughts. You realize that you are not your thoughts, and that your ruminating and spinning stories may be unrelated to what's actually going on around you. Compassion training requires you to actively work with your emotions and assumptions about yourself and others in order to release long-held resentments, hostility, and indifference. It helps you to nurture compassion, understanding, and a sense of connection with others—and to develop a deep feeling of affection for yourself. It allows you, perhaps for the very first time in your life, to be on your own side.

Charles Raison, MD, mind-body medicine researcher and professor at the University of Arizona College of Medicine, found that adolescents who went through compassion-meditation training had lower levels of inflammatory markers after a six-week program than prior to it.

In high-security prisons where inmates learned compassion meditation, violence decreased by 20 percent or more.

The most well-known form of compassion meditation—also known as *metta*, or loving-kindness—is remarkably simple and soothing. You begin with compassion toward yourself. This is important, because if you can't forgive and have compassion for yourself, you may have difficulty forgiving others.

Begin by sitting quietly, focusing on the breath. As you settle into a calm, aware state, hold an image of yourself in your mind, and begin to wish yourself well, saying this set of phrases aloud:

> May I be filled with love and kindness.
> May I be safe and protected.
> May I love and be loved.
> May I be happy and contented.
> May I be healthy and strong.
> May my life unfold with ease.

As you repeat each statement, really take it into your own heart.

Next, move your focus to someone you love dearly. Hold that person in your mind's eye and go through the phases again:

> May you be filled with love and kindness.
> May you be safe and protected.
> May you love and be loved.
> May you be happy and contented.
> May you be healthy and strong.
> May your life unfold with ease.

Next, bring to mind someone you don't know well—like the local postmaster or the person who cuts your hair. Go through the phrases again.

Next, bring into your mind's eye someone with whom you have had relational trouble or discord, someone who's caused you a little pain—

but don't try to focus on someone who you feel has traumatized you. Keep it safe.

Now go through the six phases again, thinking of this difficult person. Finally, extend your feelings of loving-kindness to include all beings:

> May all beings be filled with love and kindness.
> May all beings be safe and protected.
> May all beings love and be loved.
> May all beings be happy and contented.
> May all beings be healthy and strong.
> May all beings's lives unfold with ease.

As you end your loving-kindness practice, sit for a moment before opening your eyes and enjoy the calm sense of loving awareness as it washes over you.

9. Forgiveness

Loving-kindness helps you to let go of resentments toward yourself and others. Part of being a healthy adult means developing mental strategies that help to keep you from getting lost in the stories of your past.

Ultimately, all of the steps above won't mean anything if you can't learn to let go of the past, forgive, and move on.

This can seem like an impossible order. If a person we loved, who was supposed to protect us, instead inflicted Chronic Unpredictable Toxic Stress, it's going to be hard to forgive that person. It's going to be hard not to resent what that loss of security and trust has cost us.

Jack Kornfield, PhD, a Buddhist meditation teacher, psychologist, and change agent known for having brought the tenets of mindfulness and meditation to the West, has used both mindfulness meditation and psychotherapy to heal from his own trauma. He teaches the importance of forgiveness and compassion. Forgiveness, Kornfield says, is "the capacity to let go, to release the suffering, the sorrows, the burdens of the pains and betrayals of the past, and instead, to choose the mystery of love."

This doesn't mean condoning what happened in the past, or condoning anyone's behavior. Kornfield says, "It's not forgive and forget. In fact, forgiveness might also include quite understandably the resolve to protect yourself and never let this happen again." Forgiveness isn't "sentimental, or quick. You can't paper things over and smile and say, 'I forgive.' It is a deep process of the heart. And in the process, you need to honor the betrayal of yourself or others—the grief, the anger, the hurt, the fear." This, he admits, can take a long time. Indeed, he says, "when you do a forgiveness practice, you may realize that you're never going to forgive that person. And never takes a while."

Still, says Kornfield, "It is not necessary to be loyal to your suffering." We are often so loyal to our suffering, our regrets, our losses, focusing "on the trauma of 'what happened to me.' Yes, it happened. Yes, it was horrible. But is that what defines you?" Without forgiveness, life would be unbearable, he says. "It's hard to imagine a world without forgiveness, because we would be chained to the suffering of the past and have only to repeat it over and over again. There would be no release."

Forgiveness is not something we do just for the other person. We forgive so that we can live free of the acute suffering that comes with holding on to our past. In other words, Kornfield says, forgiveness is "for your own capacity to fulfill your life."

You can use mindfulness, loving-kindness, and guided imagery practices to help. One of my favorite forgiveness practices is a four-step forgiveness meditation taught by James Gordon, MD, founder and director of the Center for Mind-Body Medicine in Washington, DC. Gordon has led teams of practitioners to teach mindfulness practices to children suffering from natural disasters and war trauma in struggling countries around the world.

In this practice, Gordon suggests sitting in a chair and getting into a meditative, relaxed state, breathing and relaxing, as you allow an image to come to mind of someone toward whom you feel anger or resentment. Let yourself see that person now, as if she were sitting across from you in a chair.

You don't have to start with the person who hurt you most in life, but with someone toward whom you hold some resentment. Look at that person and say to him, "I forgive you. For whatever you may have done to harm me, intentional or unintentional, I forgive you." Allow yourself to soften toward that person. Imagine him coming into your heart for a moment. Breathe in. Hold him there, in your heart, breathing in and breathing out, staying present with him, relaxing, feeling forgiveness for him, for what he did, breathing. Allow yourself to be there for a minute or two or more. Now let him go, saying, "I forgive you."

In between each of these steps, sit for a moment, breathing in and out, relaxing for a few minutes.

Next, repeat this process with someone whom you have hurt in some way. Imagine her as if she were sitting in a chair across from you. Look at her and say, "Forgive me for whatever I may have done to harm you, intentionally or unintentionally; forgive me." Imagine your hearts melting together, as you hold her in your heart and mind for a few minutes. Breathe in and out, feeling forgiveness flow from her toward you. Now let her go, thanking her for the forgiveness she's offering you. Allow yourself to feel the connection between the two of you.

After breathing in and out for a few minutes, bring your own image to mind. Imagine that you're sitting in a chair across from yourself. Look at yourself and say, "I forgive you for whatever you feel you've done to hurt yourself; for however you've let yourself down, I forgive you." Feel the sensation of opening your heart to yourself, feeling the connection between you and the image of yourself sitting in a chair across from you, the connection between your hearts. Stay with that, breathing for a few more moments.

Finally, allow the feeling of forgiveness to spread from you, from your heart, to all those on the planet who are in need of forgiveness. Allow this feeling to grow and expand, breathing in, breathing out, relaxing. Say to yourself and to everyone on the planet who needs forgiveness, "I forgive you." Slowly, come back to a sense of awareness of yourself in your chair, your feet on the floor, as you breathe in and out. When you're ready, open your eyes. Enjoy the feeling of relaxation, of letting go, that comes.

A practice like this isn't a quick Band-Aid. Kornfield teaches that "Forgiveness includes all the dimensions of our life. Forgiveness is the work of the body. It's the work of the emotions. It's the work of the mind." Forgiveness involves "a shift of identity" in which you tap into your "undying capacity for love and freedom that is untouched by what happens to you."

Ultimately, your have to be ready to let go of what was in order to create the life you've always wanted.

You have to forgive, for *you*.

10. Mending the Body, Moving the Body
As we work with the mind and brain, we can't ignore the importance of working with the body, which often has been storing up physical and muscular tension from a fight, flight, or freeze state of mind for a lifetime. The following approaches are particularly good at helping to release stored up muscular tension and tame the inflammatory response.

YOGA
PET scans show that after practicing yoga, cerebral blood flow to the amygdala, the brain's alarm center, decreases, while blood flow to the frontal lobe and prefrontal cortex increases. These areas of the brain go offline during early adversity and need to be coaxed back online. Practicing yoga also increases levels of GABA—or gamma-aminobutyric acid—a chemical that improves brain function and promotes calm.

When you don't have enough GABA, you're more prone to depression and anxiety. Those who regularly practice yoga show dramatically lower levels of inflammatory biomarkers, even during lab stress tests.

TRAUMA RELEASE EXERCISES

Another benefit of yoga comes through practicing specific poses that help release tension in a muscle called the psoas, otherwise known as the "fight-or-flight muscle." Psoas muscles connect the lumbar spine to the legs, and they support our internal organs. When you feel a sudden sense of fear, worry, or loss, the psoas fire up in order to help us get ready to fight, kick, or strike out. Children who have experienced Adverse Childhood Experiences often have psoas that are tightly wound, like an animal bracing to be attacked, always in fight-or-flight mode. Over time, that tight feeling becomes so normal that we can't even tell we're holding on to emotions from our past.

David Bercelli, PhD, developed the six Trauma Release Exercises to help individuals release the muscle tension stored as a result of stress, adversity, and early trauma. That release evokes a muscular shaking process—called neurogenic tremors—which releases deep, chronic muscular tension held within the body's core. When shaking is evoked at the center of the body—an area protected by the psoas—it reverberates throughout the entire body, traveling along the spine, releasing deep chronic tension from the sacrum to the cranium.

Mary began learning TRE when she happened to meet the founder in the yoga studio where she was practicing. "The first time I tried Trauma Release Exercises, I triggered a deep shaking and trembling. My legs just shook and it went on and on." As Mary felt her body release so much pent-up energy, she realized "that when I was a kid, and I was afraid, I couldn't shake; I couldn't let my father see that I was afraid of him or I would have been humiliated for that. So I learned to contain it. In the same way that I never cried when I was a kid, because no one was going to comfort me, I never even allowed myself to tremble."

As Mary learned to discharge that tension through TRE and yoga, she felt herself "moving toward life. Like the flowers growing between the cracks in the sidewalk." Over time, she says, "I've become able to process most things without freaking out because I've learned, through practicing body movement, the art of self-soothing. This is the gift that I've been able to give myself." As a result, "I'm physically better now." Her irritable bowel syndrome and excruciating lower back pain are gone. And although the permanent changes in her skin pigmentation from her autoimmune vitiligo remain, the disease has stopped progressing. "My suicidal depression and anxiety are gone, too," she says. "I see what is good in me, and how a lot of my gifts in life—my ability to be so caring and nurturing to others—came out of my early adversity. As I've learned to shift out of that trauma state and into release, my body has changed." These days, Mary says, "I hardly ever get sick. I haven't even had a cold for four years."

BODYWORK

Bernie Siegel, MD, tells this story about the power of bodywork to bring up and release wounds from childhood that we've stored within. Siegel's own birth was traumatizing for his mother. For health reasons, she could not risk undergoing a cesarean. The labor was so difficult and prolonged that by the time he was born, his mother later told him, "They didn't hand me a baby, they handed me a purple melon." His head was misshapen; his skin, mottled. His parents "hid him away from people." But Siegel's grandmother would rub oil on and vigorously massage her newborn grandson's "purple head" several times a day to help restore his appearance. In her hands, Bernie felt deeply loved.

Fast-forward fifty years. Siegel, who has a shaved head, would occasionally get full therapeutic body massages. On one visit, his regular massage therapist wasn't available so he saw his therapist's wife. Siegel closed his eyes, anticipating a relaxing massage. This new therapist oiled her soft, female hands and began to rub his bare head. The next thing Siegel knew, he lost his sense of consciousness—something that had never happened before in his male massage therapist's hands.

When Siegel returned to consciousness, he opened his eyes to find himself surrounded by people panicking. "We couldn't communicate with you! We thought you had a stroke!" they told him. But, Siegel explains, "I knew exactly what had happened. I had become that traumatized infant again." That moment brought forth his stored traumatic body memories, only this time, as an adult who had already done a great deal of self-healing, he was able to move through those previously submerged emotions and emerge in a safe way. As a physician he knew that untouched babies don't gain weight and develop as well as babies who are massaged and touched. He felt a new gratitude for his grandmother's loving touch, and how it had helped him to heal and thrive. The pain from that early trauma was gone.

Although we do not have scientific evidence as to how and why bodywork helps with healing, these modalities have been life-changing for many individuals interviewed in these pages.

In the practice of Massage Rho, a therapist has the client guide the therapist's hands to the part of the client's body where the client feels pain. The therapist applies pressure in that area with her hands to allow deep-tissue muscle release, often releasing stored emotions as well. In Core Energetic massage, therapists release muscle tension and energy blockages that we're holding in our bodies so that feelings can be expressed. In Therapeutic Touch, a therapist trained to be sensitive to the client's energy field works with that field without ever touching the patient. Other such modalities include Reiki, shiatsu massage, and cranialsacral work.

Whatever modality you choose, the important thing is to find a practitioner-client relationship in which you feel safe.

Mary felt that she was aided in her healing by bodywork with a "medical intuitive energetic healer."

"My physical sensations would shift ten minutes into a session," she recalls. "I'd experience a complete break from the tremendous sense of anxiety that I always held inside." This break was a gift. "My medical intuitive healer was able to put me in a peaceful, healing, trusting place—in a way that I could not get to on my own. I was able to relax and feel physically safe in someone's hands for the first time in my life." After her sessions, when fears and worries would intrude again, Mary would reinvite "that sensation of being safe in someone's hands, and bring that sense of peace into moments when I came up against triggers in the real world. I internalized that feeling of being soothed and at peace with the world."

In Laura's search for healing, she has tried both Massage Rho and Core Energetic healing. Both have stirred up memories that are "known but not remembered." In one session, she says, my therapist was working around my diaphragm and I suddenly found myself screaming out loud, 'Please don't do this to me, please stop!' as I sobbed and kicked my legs like a toddler. I felt utterly powerless, and afraid, and then the feeling began to dissipate. Another time, my therapist was working on my stomach and I found myself screaming and crying, 'I can't take this weight! Please don't put this weight on me!' I felt all that weight of having to care for my mother and be the only grown-up in my adolescent world." Over the course of many sessions, the pain of the past has begun to lessen. Mary feels a sense of "letting go."

11. Managing the Mind Through the Gut

Cell for cell, we're largely made up of bacteria. In fact, single-celled organisms, mostly bacteria, outnumber our own cells ten to one. Many of these live in our gut. This gut "microbiome" determines the state of our digestive health, and influences the state of our brain. When you are under stress, the bacterial communities in your intestine become less diverse, allowing greater numbers of harmful bacteria to take over. Disorders of the gut such as irritable bowel and inflammatory bowel diseases are exacerbated by stress. Recent science shows that a sophisticated neural network transmits messages from those trillions of digestive bacteria to the brain, exerting a powerful influence on our state of mind—creating a feedback loop between the brain and the gut that goes both ways. Emotional adversity, mental stress, and trauma lead to a greater proliferation of bad bacteria in the gut, and bad bugs in the gut lead to lower mood, anxiety, depression, and a proclivity for being less resilient in the face of adversity and stress.

There are two main reasons for this. First, gut bacteria manufacture more than 80 percent of the body's supply of serotonin, which significantly influences mood. And second, good gut microbiota such as those found in probiotics have a direct effect on neurotransmitter receptors in the brain, such as GABA. Mice given probiotics had lower levels of stress-induced hormones, less anxiety, and less depression-related behavior.

And guess how the messages between the bacteria exposed to the gut and the brain were transmitted? Via the vagus nerve—which is a primary mediator of the inflammatory stress response. That's why scientists have begun to refer to our gut as "the second brain." The gut microbiome heavily influences neural development, brain chemistry, emotional behavior, pain perception, learning, and memory. Some organisms in the gut might prove useful in treatments of stress-related disorders such as anxiety and depression.

According to gastroenterologist Emeran Mayer, MD, PhD, director of the Center for Neurobiology of Stress at the University of California, Los Angeles, given the gut's multifaceted ability to communicate with the brain, "it's almost unthinkable that the gut is not playing a critical role in mind states."

Improving our diet and reducing our intake of processed foods and sugar, and adding in greens, fruits, and fermented foods rich in probiotics can play a critical role in healing the gut. This, in turn, can help patients who've suffered from early trauma to heal both body and brain.

Because microorganisms in our gut control our brain, we need to do whatever we can to make our microbiome healthy, and give the pathways in our brain all the serotonin and nutrients they need to send the correct messages along our brain's synapses. Why would you eat in a way that makes stress receptors more reactive when you are busy doing everything else you can to heal?

A number of the individuals we've followed in these pages have used nutrition to promote healing. Ellie has used diet to reduce her autoimmune psoriasis, depression, and anxiety. She switched out processed foods and sugar for leafy greens, vegetables, and fruits. At first, she noticed that during the day "my brain fog went away." Then, she says, within a few months' time, "I began to experience less anxiety. The suicidal ideation went away. I had the sense that I was becoming a more optimistic person. The shift was subtle, but it was there. I felt as if I was transforming my mind and body with food." Then Ellie noticed another improvement: "I began to feel good when I woke up in the morning," she says. "My whole life I'd claimed I wasn't a morning person, and it was the best I could do to get up by ten or eleven. But one day I got up out of bed at 7:30 a.m. I noticed the sound of the birds chirping outside my window. I felt as if a twenty-pound weight had been lifted off my shoulders. That's when it hit me: I was awake, alert, alive."

Her autoimmune psoriasis decreased. "My skin became clear for the first time in years."

Ellie decided to become a licensed holistic health nutritionist and coach. "I feel that, no matter what our story might be, by addressing the gut-mind connection and working to change our microbiome in our gut, we can help to rewrite the story of our physical and mental well-being."

Kendall has used diet to help regrow the lining of her gut, after a lifetime of celiac disease. John also found that diet helped him become healthier. Kat, too, found that when she began to "heal the gut," she began to slowly help heal her mind. "I realized that my gut was the thing that all my life I had trouble listening to, from that very first moment in the station wagon when I was five, and I knew something bad had happened to my mom, but I told myself that all was well. It made sense to me that now I needed to pay attention to what my gut needed to heal itself." Kat cleaned up her diet, cutting out foods that her immune system might be reacting to, including dairy, gluten, sugar, and processed carbohydrates, all of which can contribute to the buildup of bad bacteria. She added in "fermented kimchi, sauerkraut, and probiotics" to help build up the good bacteria in her gut. "It took six months," she says, to see a real difference in how she felt, but "working with a nutritionist and changing my diet was one of the most helpful things I did in my journey to heal."

With all her efforts at finding wholeness, Kat feels that "I'm finally rewriting the script of my past. I can look back now and say I'm truly grateful for everything that has played a part in my story and in who I am now. I'm rewriting my story by giving it meaning, and in helping others to do the same in my work now as a life coach."

Kat likes to think "that people see me and are able to say to themselves, 'Here is somebody who rewrote the story of her brain, her body, her relationships, and her life.' If I, after having been through what I have been through, can turn a traumatic life into a joyful life, well, they can find healing, too."

12. Only Connect

We often develop wounds from relationships, but we also heal in relationship to each other. When we are in healthy interactions and supportive relationships, when we feel "tended and befriended," our bodies and brains have a better chance of healing, too. For instance, having strong social ties helps to improve outcomes for women with breast cancer, multiple sclerosis, and other diseases. In part, that's because positive, supportive interactions help us to produce more oxytocin, a "feel-good" hormone that helps to mediate and dial down the overactive inflammatory stress response.

It's important to know that you are not alone in your feelings of loss, shame, guilt, anxiety, or grief. When you reach out to others who understand the fallout from Post Childhood Adversity Syndrome, you gain not only support but life perspective. You see that your own story is one of many stories that make up the larger hurt of humanity.

And when you begin to understand that your pain is not just your pain, but is shared by so many others—at least 64 percent of the people around you carry a history of adversity that may affect their adult health—you can begin to share support and ideas for healing. You can find ways to start right where you are, no matter where you find yourself now.

That might mean joining a community mindfulness meditation group, MBSR class, or reaching out to friends with whom you enjoy healthy, caring relationships, and who are willing to share their own stories and resources that they've found to be helpful. It may mean passing along the Adverse Childhood Experiences questionnaire, or even this book, to family members, friends, or coworkers whom you feel would be helped by it, and using it as a way to jump-start a deeper, more honest conversation.

CHAPTER SEVEN

Seeking Professional Help
to Heal from Post Childhood
Adversity Syndrome

Sometimes, you cannot heal on your own, despite your best efforts. You need the help of a well-trained professional.

1. Therapy Matters

According to Jack Kornfield, PhD, psychologist and meditation teacher, there are times when we need to bring unresolved issues into a therapeutic relationship, and have help in unpacking the past. Even "meditation is not always enough," he says. Kornfield grew up with "the pain of living in a family with a violent and abusive father, and the underlying fear" that comes with such a childhood. Many teachers and students who come to meditation hold "a great deal of unresolved grief, fear, woundedness, and unfinished business from the past," he says. Even meditation teachers can find that despite years of deep practice, "major areas of our beings are unconscious, fearful, or disconnected" and they are in need of "psychotherapy in order to deal with these issues." There are, says Kornfield, times when we need to get help from "a deep and therapeutic relationship." Kornfield found that he needed to combine his meditation practice with working with "a skilled therapist who would call my attention to movements or emotions that were unconscious to me."

When you are in a therapeutic relationship with a skilled therapist and experience something "old," that memory is paired with the positive experience of being seen by someone who attunes to you, sees you, and accepts you just as you are, whatever your experience was—and you begin to heal. When you begin to feel trust, perhaps for the first time in your life, and when this process is repeated, you modify old circuits in the brain that tell you that you cannot trust. You create new brain cells and connections that allow you to create new habits and responses to other people. Indeed, part of the power of therapy is that one can learn, finally, as an adult, to become attached to a safe person. You can begin to feel safe in engaging, interacting, and bonding in a relationship. In this way, a therapist's unconditional acceptance rewires you so that you have a more fully formed, healthier sense of self.

Therapy can also heal the underlying, cellular damage of traumatic stress on DNA. Trauma patients show higher levels of damage to their DNA, but therapy actually changes the integrity of DNA at the molecular level, even repairing DNA. In one study, these changes remained in individuals even a year after their therapy ended.

A fifty-eight-year-old patient of Dr. Vincent Felitti's, whose story remains anonymous in his work, but whom I refer to here as "Alice," discovered the role that her childhood ACEs played in her lifelong physical and emotional pain—and the power of the therapeutic process. She writes that she was a thin, compliant child with many health problems. She recalled only small bits of her childhood: being spanked when she was seven, sleeping with a baseball bat beside her bed, and being ill with frequent infections that dumbfounded her pediatrician, who also worried over why her lips and fingernails often turned blue.

Surgeons removed her tonsils and adenoids, and irradiated her thymus. At the age of twelve, Alice developed a heart murmur that her doctor could "hear without a stethoscope." Over the next thirty years, she endured a severe pelvic inflammatory infection, breast infections, intense pain in her pelvic area, anxiety, depression, and suicidal ideation. She often felt spacey and jumpy.

Alice later married and divorced, and while rearing two small children alone, wanted to become healthier for her children's sake. She decided to look for why she had "extensive childhood amnesia" and always felt "so miserable." She saw a therapist, and told him of a nightmare that plagued her, "the sounds of the clink of a belt buckle and the zip of a zipper." After many sessions, Alice's therapist guided her to find her distraught seven-year-old self and talk to her about that day when she was spanked. Alice relived the pain and terror of the event; over the course of therapy she realized that it was her grandfather who had harmed her, and filled in many of the blank places in her childhood. In a safe, therapeutic environment, with a skilled professional, she began to feel the security she never felt as a child and to heal.

When she went to her next annual cardiology examination, Alice's doctor told her that her heart murmur was gone. As she remembered the origin of her pain, her physical pain and illness improved.

2. Somatic Experiencing

When kids face adversity and trauma, they employ defensive fight-or-flight strategies or go into a "freeze" state, where they have little sense of what they are feeling in their body. In working with patients who have faced childhood adversity and trauma, psychologists try to bring their feelings back online at a pace that's comfortable for them, so that they can recognize and manage what they are feeling. One of the best ways to achieve this is through a therapeutic practice known as Somatic Experiencing, or SE—which helps you to focus on the sensations you perceive in your body.

Somatic Experiencing was developed by Peter A. Levine, PhD, director of the Somatic Experiencing Trauma Institute. He noticed that animals in the wild rebound from life-threatening situations after being immobilized by fear. When that threat passes, they spontaneously discharge all the physical tension they had been holding inside during that fight, flight, or freeze state by involuntarily shaking or trembling. This physical expenditure of energy, this release, triggers a reset in their breathing pattern so that they begin to breathe more deeply again, which resets their autonomic nervous system back to normal, restoring their body to a state of equilibrium. They come back to center. The fear is gone, and so is all the excess energy that came from holding that fear and tension inside their body. They can move on.

Somatic Experiencing allows us a safe way to discharge all the emotions and sensations we've stored during traumatic events so that we can begin to heal. Trained practitioners utilize Somatic Experiencing to help alleviate the symptoms of mental and physical trauma-related health problems, including those that stem from Post Childhood Adversity Syndrome, developmental trauma, shock trauma, and post-traumatic stress disorder.

Clients aren't asked to talk about their traumatic experiences—but to learn about how the body regulates stress and to take note of their physical sensations, to tune in to them and see what feelings, thoughts, and images arise. Slowly, in an environment of safety, individuals learn to experience small amounts of that original distress and release that stored energy, which in turn allows their nervous system to return to balance. Over time, more and more of an individual's most difficult emotions can begin to surface safely.

In order to handle the physical sensations and memories that arise, individuals learn a process called "pendulation." They establish a "safe place" in their mind—a touch point that they can go to anytime to feel secure. This might be the memory of someone close to them or a benefactor who helped them, or a safe place they've been to or imagined, often in nature. Or they might simply hold an object that helps to ground them in the present moment.

Clients pendulate back and forth between their safe place and the more difficult physical sensations and emotions that arise from past adversity and trauma; they learn to safely face and discharge that early stress so that their nervous system can return to a balanced state. Levine calls this "the rhythm of contraction and extraction."

Pendulating also soothes while discharging that state of stress-reactive arousal. You might discharge your traumatic sensations in tears or sobbing, even shaking, before you come back to your safe place and arrive in a moment where you can breathe easily again—a key sign that your autonomic nervous system is calming down and healing.

As you learn to do this, you increase your zone of tolerance so that you can handle a little more wobble in your life.

For Georgia, who grew up with a controlling mother and an angry father, and was so sensitive she picked up on tension in her home "before arguments even happened," somatic experiencing allowed her to move to a new level of healing despite the trauma of her early life with her parents, her chronic health problems, and the trauma of multiple back surgeries. "I needed what I thought of as an 'emotional rehab' plan. I either had to get on a journey of healing or just fold it all up."

Georgia began with mindfulness meditation, which had a powerful effect, but she also needed one-on-one guidance to help her reconnect with her body and her emotions, so she began Somatic Experiencing Therapy. Once a week, for more than a year, Georgia met with an SE therapist. She says, "My therapist helped me to realize how my body makes its noise. There were times when my therapist would look at a subtle reaction I wasn't even aware I was having and ask me, 'What just happened?' If I said, 'I don't know what you mean,' she'd ask me to pause. I'd realize that I was holding back tears. When I said, 'I feel sad,' she'd ask me, 'Where?' My sadness often started with a sharp pain under my shoulder blade. If I didn't allow the grief to be there and let it come up—usually in tears—the pain would radiate way down my back. It wouldn't go away if I didn't listen to it." Other times, Georgia felt discomfort in her stomach and abdominal area. Her therapist helped her to focus her attention on the physical and emotional pain she was holding on to so tightly in the core of her body.

Georgia uses the skills she learned through somatic experiencing in her day-to-day life to help her to manage her emotional pain and physical illness. "If my emotions are very intense, I deal with them in small steps, finding a place of comfort, and then dealing with whatever feels painful a little bit more.

"If I feel sad, I start to tune in and have a conversation with my body, and ask it what it needs. I've learned to listen to the pain in my shoulder, or my GI symptoms—my 'gut feelings'—when the sensation starts, rather than wait until it knocks me off my feet."

She's also learned how to self-soothe throughout her day. "When you have been on the achievement superhighway all of your life, it's difficult to step back, even when you are in pain, and create moments of comfort for yourself. But I'm learning the art of comfort, caring enough about myself to take a moment to sit on the front porch in the sun with a cup of tea, to go on the walk I've been meaning to take all day, or just lie down and enjoy the wash of good pleasure hormones that come with snuggling with my rescue mutt."

Georgia has learned "to use my voice to speak so that my body doesn't have to." She's also been able to establish boundaries with her narcissistic mother and tell her, "I need you to stop." She's moved away from toxic relationships and friendships. "I've learned, by listening to my body, what people, interactions, and pressures make me reexperience that old, toxic sense of survival-based arousal."

Somatic experiencing helps someone who has experienced trauma to slow down, experience painful sensations comfortably, and to tolerate feelings without getting overwhelmed by them. When you feel safe enough to be aware of your feeling state, you can regulate your emotions and actions.

Somatic exercises also help you to recognize when you're primed to erupt with anger or anxiety, overreact, lose your cool, and say and do things you don't mean. You can learn to "hear" the signs that you are on your edge: exhibited by muscle tension, a "pain in the neck," forgetting to breathe, pain, numbness, bodily discomfort, or fluish fatigue. You learn to pause and center yourself before you react in ways you might later regret.

3. Guided Imagery, Creative Visualization, and Hypnosis

Guided visualizations use your imagination and imagery to change your neural structure. When you engage in guided imagery, you use the right hemisphere of the brain, which is responsible for mental processing, to rewire old patterns.

"Mental imagery is not the same thing as just thinking about something," says Bernie Siegel, MD. Analytical thinking "happens mostly in regions on the left side of the brain, where language, planning, judgment, and numbers reign. Creative visualization, or mental imagery, is a process that engages mostly the right side; it involves using the visual, auditory, and olfactory senses, as well as memory, mood, emotions."

To really grasp how these two sides of the brain work differently, try the lemon experiment. Think about putting lemons on your shopping list. Just that thought—"I need to buy some lemons" activated the left side of your brain. Now, imagine that lemons are selling for $1.99 a pound at the store. Thinking about buying the lemons and paying for them— that's all left-brain activity helping you to get done what you need to do.

Now, imagine holding a ripe, fresh lemon in your hand. Feel "the waxy surface of the rind against your fingers, and smell the warm citrus aroma," says Siegel. "Imagine that you take a sharp knife and slice the lemon into quarters. Some of the juice sprays out and the lemony aroma becomes even stronger. Place one of the lemon quarters between your thumb and fingers and squeeze gently. Watch as the beads of juice rise up and trickle down the moist, plump flesh of the fruit. Raise the lemon to your mouth and let the juice trickle down to the back of your tongue."

By now, you are experiencing the lemon on an entirely different level, with your whole brain. You are salivating and the bitterness of the lemon makes you shudder or pucker your lips. Your body responds as if it were tasting a real lemon. Visualization convinced your brain that the lemon was real.

Athletes use creative visualization to enhance their performance by imagining swinging the bat or dunking the ball before the big game. If an individual practices a five-finger piano exercise every day merely in his imagination, he shows as much neural growth in the corresponding motor cortex of the brain as do those who actually practiced that same exercise daily on the piano. Mental imagery fools the brain into believing we are actually doing the thing we are imagining.

Even patients who took placebo pills and who were *told* the pills were placebo reported less pain than patients who received no treatment. It may be that, when we're given a message, even if we know that what we're being told isn't "real," that message nevertheless creates a kind of "bodily memory" within us—one that initiates physical and neurobiological changes. This is a pretty good explanation for how and why creative visualization and hypnosis work, as well.

In Laura's healing journey, she has learned through guided imagery to call upon a "Wise Self" who comes back and gives the wounded, abandoned young girl she once was the soothing and acceptance she never got from the mom who made a pastime of humiliating her. "I imagine my Wise Self as being about sixty years old. She is wearing my same big, round tortoiseshell glasses, and her long dark brown hair has a sharp streak of gray. She is smiling, just smiling this warm, healing smile at me, as if she loves me unconditionally, the way a mother loves a child. When I'm feeling really sad, or stressed, I imagine her sitting beside me, holding me and saying, "It's okay, sweetheart, it's okay; this too, will be okay, really, you'll see." Almost instantaneously, says Laura, "I feel calmed, the way you might if you were ten and you were in your mother's arms, and your mom was that wise, it's-going-to-be-okay, I-love-you-no-matter-what kind of mom. The mom I didn't have."

Michele, at thirteen, suffered an allergic reaction to the antibiotic that her doctor prescribed for an infection, causing a rare, life-threatening condition so severe that she was treated as a trauma burn victim. Unable to bear the pain and shock of the sudden medical trauma, her thirteen-year-old brain went offline. She recovered physically but was trapped in a state of perpetual anxiety, feeling that she was "walking around in a body that could betray me any second." Michele refused to talk to her doctors or therapists about what happened to her. She went silent. She was too afraid to feel any more pain.

Twenty years later, by her midthirties, Michele was riddled with chronic fatigue, irritable bowel syndrome, chronic sinus infections, anxiety and depression, and muscle spasms, among other problems. In order to get free of the fear that always gripped her and reclaim her power over the past, she decided to record her story. As Michele wrote, and brought up her pain-embedded memories of that time, she says, "My hair fell out; I developed a three-inch bald spot."

Writing helped her feel a little better, but she still felt stuck. "Despite my best efforts, I could not kick the habit of anxiety," she says. "I felt like I had a trauma addiction. I could not let go of my fear. My mind just kept going back to my trauma; I had latched on to the anxiety I'd felt when I was thirteen, and I couldn't let go of it. I couldn't quit my fear habit."

Then one day Michele was driving and "heard someone talking about kicking a nicotine habit with hypnosis. I didn't believe in hypnosis," but she also recognized "that I had done all of the traditional therapy I wanted to do. I no longer wanted to talk about what had happened to me. Retelling the story in talk therapy hadn't brought me the sense of freedom I'd hoped to find." Perhaps hypnosis could help her recover without having to verbalize her memories again.

Michele interviewed seven hypnotherapists and found one with neuroscience-based therapeutic training. That first session her hypnotist talked her through a relaxation process, and then asked her to visualize being in a room with no roof, in which two chairs faced each other. "She asked me to sit down in one of the chairs, and to place a box that had a red helium balloon attached to it in the chair facing me. She guided me through the process of putting all of the fear related to my illness, all of my anger, sadness, all of my negative and disturbing emotions, my terror and anxiety of what happened when I was thirteen in that box. When the box was full, I closed it and let it lift up through the open roof. I watched it float away."

Then Michele's hynpotherapist asked her to imagine seeing herself sitting in the chair opposite her. She told her, "You are facing yourself and I want you to look at you and forgive you for all the negative emotions you have felt about your illness. Forgive yourself for the pain and terror and fear. Forgive yourself for the sadness and illness and all the sicknesses. Forgive yourself for not being able to find a way to let it go." This process of self-forgiveness continued, until her hypnotist said, "hug yourself, tight, and then let yourself shrink down to an inch and land in your heart." As she said these words, Michele's hypnotherapist tapped her on her arm.

Michele recalls feeling "disappointingly awake the whole time." But when the session ended and she opened her eyes, she was surprised to find herself feeling "groggy, as if I were waking from a nap." She assumed she had been "visualizing for about fifteen minutes—but it turned out to have been almost an hour.

"I went to bed that night annoyed, feeling I'd just wasted money and time," she says. "But that was the first night I slept straight through for eight hours since my illness. The next day I woke up and for the first time that I could remember I felt no anxiety, I felt no fear. Five days later I was still feeling calm. I thought, 'Something must be wrong here, I just feel so good, this can't be right.'"

Six hypnosis sessions later, Michele says, "I was changed. My emotional state was completely different. I was sleeping again, I was relaxed. I felt happy. My mom made a comment that I'll never forget. She said, 'Michele, you have a real laugh again, the same laugh that you had when you were thirteen and healthy, before you went into that hospital. Ever since then, your laugh has sounded faked and forced. This is your real laugh; this is the real you."

Feeling freed from her persistent, free-floating anxiety, Michele awakened in other ways as well. Around the time she had started hypnosis she had also started ballroom dancing, which helps her to continue to "wake up to joy." She's also launched an active blog for those who've suffered life-altering trauma. And Michele is now a certified professional coach specializing in post-traumatic stress disorder and a certified hypnotist.

"Our subconscious mind is 88 percent of our mind, and I think that was the part of my brain that hypnosis spoke to," she says.

As Michele's symptoms of anxiety disappeared, so did her physical illnesses. "My liver enzymes had been high for years and suddenly, they normalized. My irritable bowel resolved. The pain in my muscles just went away." Most remarkably, Michele's osteoporosis reversed itself. Her body was in a new state of relaxation. She also relied on good nutrition and did a diligent strength-training program. "My bones are strong and healthy, now," she says.

Michele wrote her story from a place of healing, calling it *Before the World Intruded: Conquering the Past and Creating the Future*. She also started her own radio show and interviewed experts on trauma, PTSD, and healing. "I've gone from the girl who couldn't talk about trauma to the woman who talks for healing," she says, laughing.

It doesn't mean that life is trouble-free now, she says. "But I've learned to cope with what comes. And I've learned to stop asking, 'Why did this happen to me?' That question takes you down a dark rabbit hole. The real question is 'What can I do with what happened to me?' It is so easy to lose hope, and you can never lose hope. You can always make meaning come out of what happened to you. You can always find something that will work for you to help you heal."

4. Neurofeedback

Electroencephalographic (EEG) Neurofeedback improves brain functioning. According to neuroscientist Ruth Lanius, MD, PhD, director of the post-traumatic stress disorder (PTSD) research unit at the University of Western Ontario in Canada, "Neurofeedback can help to bring some of the brain networks that are interrupted by trauma back online."

In EEG Neurofeedback, patients sit in a chair facing a laptop screen. The laptop is connected to electrodes on their scalp to monitor their brain's electrical activity. Computer software monitors brain wave patterns—and lets them know how well they are managing their brain states by changing the images they see on the screen.

For instance, the computer might show you the image of a field. When your brain is underactivated in a key area, the field, which is constantly changing in response to your brain's activity, may appear to you to be muddy and gray, the flowers wilted. But when that area of the brain starts to come back online, it triggers the field to burst into color, with blooming flowers and a sound track of birds singing. In this way, EEG Neurofeedback gives individuals real-time feedback about what their brain is doing, and how they're feeling, enabling them to learn to reliably influence their own neuronal activity. With practice, people learn how to activate certain thought patterns that lead to the neural activity that is associated with pleasant images and sounds.

You might think of the EEG Neurofeedback process as acting as a conductor, trying to get different parts of the orchestra to play a little more softly in some cases, and a little louder in others, in order to achieve greater synchronicity and harmony. After a neurofeedback session, patients show greater network connectivity in a significant number of brain areas and show improved ability to rebound emotionally.

If you do look for a therapist licensed in EEG Neurofeedback, ask what the therapist's experience is in helping individuals with early adversity and trauma.

5. EMDR and Desensitizing Memory

Certain forms of therapy work by helping individuals to remember difficult experiences safely and to learn to relate to those memories in ways that no longer cause pain in the present. By going through controlled exposure and reexposure, they learn not to associate negative emotions with objects or memories that they fear. Through working with a therapist to do this in a safe manner, they gradually become able to bring to mind an object, person, or event so that it no longer fills them with dread. They become free.

Danielle Schiller, PhD, assistant professor of neuroscience and psychiatry at Mount Sinai, has found through her research that "If you present a negative memory over and over again, without anything bad happening, it is possible for most people to overcome their fear. You will still know what happened, and the information will be available to you," says Schiller. "But the emotion will be gone." For instance, it may become possible to be around a parent who humiliated or harmed you, and over time, no longer experience waves of panic and anxiety. The fear is no longer there.

By helping to uncouple fear from what is remembered, it may indeed be possible to untether ourselves from our most painful emotional memories.

EMDR, or Eye Movement Desensitization and Reprocessing, is a potent form of psychotherapy that helps with this process. EMDR therapy was developed by Francine Shapiro, PhD, senior research fellow at the Mental Research Institute in Palo Alto, California, in 1990. Shapiro noticed that if an individual shifted his gaze back and forth quickly, as we do in the deepest stages of our REM, or rapid eye movement sleep, while thinking about painful past experiences, the emotions and stress reactions associated with those memories would dissipate.

As a psychologist, Shapiro realized that "many patients might come in to see a physician or psychiatrist complaining of anxiety, but if the patient wasn't reporting PTSD or major trauma, the clinician or therapist might never know about their early history of adversity." This seemed to Shapiro to be a very big miss. Like Ruth Lanius, Shapiro found that "adverse experiences cause many of the same symptoms of PTSD—but lead to an even wider range of emotional and physical symptoms than major trauma. Yet if patients don't talk about them, and they don't fit into the PTSD category, psychiatrists don't know, and so they treat those symptoms as anxiety and prescribe medication."

But medication doesn't help us to revise how we respond to our memories; it masks the anxiety that has shadowed us into the present.

To Shapiro, therapists needed to look "more closely at the kinds of ubiquitous adverse experiences that most people have had, the smaller traumas" and how these unprocessed memories might be "behind many of the disorders we see."

For instance, says Shapiro, if we read the following list of negative beliefs and find that any of these statements give us an uncomfortable feeling in our body, or cause our breath to quicken, shorten, or catch, we probably have unprocessed emotions from earlier life events. Some of the negative beliefs we might be carrying around include these:

> I don't deserve love.
> I am terrible.
> I am a bad person.
> I am inadequate.

I am not good enough.

I am ugly (my body is hateful).

I do not deserve . . .

I am stupid (not smart enough).

I am a disappointment.

I deserve to die.

I deserve to be miserable.

I am different (don't belong).

I should have done something.

I did something wrong.

I should have known better.

Shapiro found that she could help patients to safely tap into their negative emotions and reprocess early memories associated with their negative, emotionally damaging beliefs by working with the body's natural process of rapid eye movement.

Here's how this reprocessing works: in an EMDR therapy session, a patient is helped to cue into painful emotions. As those emotions lead them to recall specific difficult experiences, and deep-seated feelings about those memories arise, they are asked to shift their gaze back and forth rapidly, often by following a pattern of lights that move from right to left, right to left, in a movement that simulates REM sleep. The therapist guides the client's focus of attention.

Or, individuals can hold a small wand in each hand that pulses intermittently from right to left. Other methods include listening to bilateral tones, or bilateral tapping, or simply having a therapist hold up two fingers and asking a patient to shift their gaze from side to side. The therapist uses structured procedures to make sure the client focuses on and processes everything that needs to be addressed.

"We all have an information processing center in the brain that is geared to take in experience and bring it to resolution. We take our present experience, relate it to all of our past memories and events in our life, process this information, and make new conclusions," says Shapiro. Those conclusions often evoke intense feelings. "With EMDR, we are looking at the early memories that might be causing those feelings, the current situations that trigger those feelings, what kind of symptoms a patient has, and what's needed for the future for an individual to go forward in a healthier way."

EMDR therapy appears to link into the same neurological processes that take place in REM sleep and clean up the brain. The repetitive redirecting of attention in EMDR induces a neurobiological state similar to that in REM sleep, and this process—both in sleep and EMDR—supports the brain integration that is dysregulated during adversity and Chronic Unpredictable Toxic Stress. This integration can, in turn, lead to a reduction in the episodic memories of traumatic events that we store in the hippocampus, and downshift the amygdala's alert state.

Other studies have shown that EMDR increases the volume of the hippocampus, which tends to be smaller in individuals who suffered early adversity and trauma.

By inducing a similar processing experience to REM sleep in a safe therapeutic setting through EMDR therapy, "we are jump-starting that process so that we can finally move to resolution, so that negative emotions are no longer there," Shapiro explains. Painful memories of adversity "are like little dream scenes that we don't want around anymore. Because they are stored in an unprocessed form, they retain an emotional charge. So they just remain that way and no amount of passing years changes them at all." But once we've "processed the old memory, it lessens an individual's level of day-to-day distress."

There is, Shapiro underscores, such "a massive amount of suffering out there, a pervasiveness of pain. It transmits from one generation to the next. And yet here we have a very effective tool to help reset the brain."

This process can work even when our memories are so old or so buried that they exist outside of our conscious awareness.

Priscilla, who nearly died when she was a child, suffered from debilitating panic attacks, and was diagnosed with the heart condition mitral valve prolapse, decided to try EMDR therapy to deal with feelings that she hadn't been able to resolve despite trying a wide range of other modalities, including fifteen years of talk therapy. With EMDR, she says, "I was able to bring up memories without having to summon them. I began to understand that my nervous system was an entity unto itself, one that could be activated, and could also be calmed down. My nervous system was simply doing what nervous systems do; it was overactivated. But most things I was trying weren't really getting to the heart of that problem."

Priscilla's therapist, Gina Colelli, had studied with Francine Shapiro, and had worked with first responders and survivors of the terrorist attack on 9/11. She had "a reputation for helping people who had hit a wall with traditional psychotherapy."

Priscilla was able to tap into her emotions, bring up memories of her past when her parents had abandoned her—and recall childhood panic attacks that she had not remembered. And as she did, she says, "I allowed those difficult feelings to pass through me until I began to feel better—alive and resilient. I was ready to leave the pain of my family behind." EMDR helped her to "see the lightness that was inside of me. And I could go out into the world radiating that light."

In the process, Priscilla came to realize that "I didn't hate my mother. I accepted her as she was. I realized that there was nothing to forgive, she was just who she was, doing the best she could do at the time." The timing for letting go of her anger and resentment toward her mother couldn't have been better—that year, Priscilla's mom deteriorated from Alzheimer's, and Priscilla was able to spend that last year of her life finding ways to connect with her before she passed away.

According to Colelli, "When we clear the nervous system, the language, emotions, and behavior that accompany them move from a subjective to an objective experience." In other words, we can observe what is happening—but we don't feel the same painful emotions. We can move on to the possibility of the full life we can have right here, right now.

EMDR may provide a way to reexperience the feelings that accompany an early Adverse Childhood Experiences memory, and intervene, to reconsolidate that memory in a way that detaches it from the overwhelming fear that we felt at the time.

Today, Shapiro's EMDR therapy has been endorsed by the World Health Organization as one of only two forms of psychotherapy for the treatment of trauma in children and adults in natural disasters and war settings.

CHAPTER EIGHT

Parenting Well When You Haven't Been Well Parented: Fourteen Strategies to Help You Help Your Children

The following strategies will help you, as a parent, teacher, or mentor, to help children and adolescents recover from the effects of childhood Chronic Unpredictable Toxic Stress.

It is never too late to help your child and your family.

A good childhood or a bad childhood doesn't hang on a single moment or even a string of them. You can still make a change and intervene.

———

According to interpersonal neurobiologist Dan Siegel, MD, there is no such thing as perfect parenting, or being a parent who does everything so wisely that our child's developing brain creates pristine neurobiological interconnections. "Understanding alone cannot prevent disrupted connections from occurring," says Siegel. "Some will inevitably happen. The challenge we all share is to embrace our humanity with humor and patience so that we can in turn relate to our children with openness and kindness. To continually chastise ourselves for our 'errors' with our children keeps us involved in our own emotional issues and out of relationship with our children."

We may not be able to protect children from all adversity and traumatic experiences. You may not be the perfect parent in every second. But you can nurture children and teens in ways that prevent chronic, unpredictable stress from taking a long-term toll. As parents and caregivers, we have the ultimate role in preventing and modulating the effect adversity has on our children.

Even when you haven't been the parent you have wanted to be, says Siegel, "It's never too late." The mind "is truly 'plastic'—changeable through experience—and it is possible at any age to move it toward greater health and harmony." Even when a parent is stressed, if things settle down, and you move into a more relaxed state and develop a strong stable environment for your child and yourself, that's okay.

Recent studies bear this out. Even rats who inherited stress biomarker proteins from their mothers didn't retain those biomarkers when the stress in their lives receded. Similarly, when a human parent suffers from a psychiatric condition, but demonstrates good parenting skills, his or her children are no more likely to develop the disease than children who have no genetic predisposition.

I have worried about this myself, since my own children, when they were very young, watched me manage a life-threatening autoimmune illness. I was hospitalized several times and was unable to see them, and I had monthlong periods of being bedridden at home. I asked Deany Laliotis, a psychotherapist in Washington, DC, who specializes in treating simple and complex traumatic stress responses, if my kids would be irreparably harmed by their experiences. Her words reassured me: "If you have come through that time together as a family and your children felt secure in their attachment to you, and if a new calm is now the family norm, the developing brain will make new, more positive associations that will over time override the old negative associations."

I hope that my kids will hold on to their newer memories of my hiking with them, baking cakes, walking and talking on the beach, and having long nighttime chats about life—and that these will replace their memories of pushing me in a wheelchair when they were six and ten, or of my gray face as I lay in a hospital bed. Memories of the mom who all but disappeared on them have, I hope, been integrated with positive memories of the mom who was always devoted to them and to their well-being.

Some of those more painful images and memories may not be gone, says Laliotis, "but what matters for the kids is how you relate to them around their experiences, and that even though life was traumatic earlier, it is stable now, before the end of childhood."

If you change how you behave, including how you react to life's stressors, you will start a new process of "childhood remembering."

The human brain has the remarkable, biologically innate capacity to break apart this early neural cement, to grow new neurons and new synaptic connections. And the younger a child is, the easier it is for the brain to adapt, which means we should help our kids as early as we can.

———

To improve your parenting, there is no more important step than learning to manage your own reactivity. But as you set out to work on yourself, you can take these small, simple steps to become more present, attuned, and empathetic and to imbue your family life with the kind of calm that ensures your child builds a balanced and healthy nervous system for life. You will give him or her the best possible chance of having the lifelong good health you want for your child.

The following fourteen tips on parenting, mentoring, and caregiving are meant to be first steps in helping you with your own parenting behavior. They are by no means all that's needed. If the adversity your child is facing is outside your control or beyond your self-control (because of your own or someone else's addiction, depression, or mental illness if there is physical or sexual abuse or unmitigating emotional abuse), you must seek professional or legal help.

1. Manage Your Own "Baggage"

Clearly, the biggest gift you can give your children is to manage your own unresolved issues, and keep them from spilling over from your childhood to pollute your children's. Interpersonal neurobiologist Dan Siegel puts it simply: "Better parents make better kids. The biggest issue in determining secure attachment for a kid is how well his or her parents have made sense of their own childhood experience." You have to learn to take care of yourself, so that you can be a good parent to your child.

"As parents we can only do the best we can," Siegel says. It's helpful to realize that you are not alone in your need to do work on yourself, in order to be more conscious in your interactions with your children. You can move from historic insecurity to a present life of security and therefore help to bring security into your child's life.

If you start to manage your own stuff so that you are less reactive, you are doing the single most important thing you can do to ameliorate, or correct, the inevitable mistakes that you will make—and that all parents make. And you will begin to make fewer of them.

Siegel calls this ability to manage your own reactivity so that you are more responsive to your child's needs "parental regulation." The more you learn to regulate your behavior as a parent, the more you'll be able to provide your kids with what they need to feel safe.

2. Don't Confuse Chronic Unpredictable Toxic Stress with Childhood Challenges that Foster Resilience

The most reliable way to raise a child to become a brave, kind, resilient, and curious adult is to ensure that when he or she is young, there is as little chronic, unpredictable stress as possible. We need to distinguish between the kind of adversity that harms and the kind that helps make children ready to hold their own in a tough world. We need to balance between protecting them and pushing them a little so that they can survive out there.

Paul Tough writes in his book *How Children Succeed* that at the same time that we want to shield our kids, we also have to provide discipline, rules, limits. Every child needs some "child-sized adversity, a chance to fall and get back up again on his own, without help." The long struggle we face as parents, Tough says, is "between our urge to provide everything for our child, to protect him from all harm, and our knowledge that if we really want him to succeed, we need to first let him fail. Or more precisely, we need to help him learn to manage failure."

Dan Siegel puts it this way: It's your job to provide a balanced approach. You lend support while supporting separation, providing a safe haven while also encouraging exploration.

While you protect your children from harm, you also want them to learn to handle adversity, deal with hardship, disappointments, losses. They need a little grit. Again, kids need to develop a sense of inner resilience in order to have wobble, in order not to be toppled by life.

On the one hand you cannot, nor should you try to, protect your kids from everything. You have to differentiate between safe and unsafe struggles. If your child is struggling with getting chores or homework problems done, or arguing with a sibling, you can support him with advice while not stepping in to take care of his problem or do his chore for him.

For instance, if your child's teacher calls your child out for turning in homework late, or not preparing for a test, or he keeps getting up late and missing the bus, he has to face the consequences, and learn from the experience. He has to dig deep and do whatever he needs to do to be prepared, catch the bus, shift his habits in ways that create the scaffolding for his own future success. You'll do little good to march in to demand why the teacher is being so hard on your child or ask if he can retake the test. You deprive your child of learning how to self-advocate and manage mild adversity, find his or her own sense of mastery, and get up and rebound from failure.

If your child says, "I left my homework in my locker and have a test tomorrow," avoid giving negative predictions ("Well, you will fail that test, won't you!") or immediate solutions ("I'll call the teacher!"). Instead, you might say, "It sounds like you have a problem. I know you can handle it. What are your options?"

Adversity in and of itself is not the problem. Adversity—and failure—are facts of human life. They are how we learn. Let your child learn competence by solving her own child-sized or teen-sized problems.

A little bit of failure and grit in the face of a challenge is a good thing, but if your child is facing bullying; struggling with a learning disability or emotional health problem; experimenting with health-risk behaviors such as sex, drugs, or alcohol; or facing emotional or physical abuse of any sort, it's your job as a parent to step in.

Moreover, when loved and trusted adults in a child's life *are* the adversity—when we confuse parental humiliation, put-downs, teasing, silent treatments, name calling, yelling and screaming, emotional and physical neglect, emotionally erratic outbursts, or fits with "toughening her up" or "making a man of him"—then *we* are our child's source of stress. Chronic, toxic criticism and humiliation are the kinds of unpredictable childhood adversity that lead to lifelong immune dysfunction and health challenges, as well as a permeating, lifelong sense of emotional loss.

Toxic stress doesn't give our kids grit; it hurts their bodies and brains, reducing their well-being for life. It doesn't make them stronger or tougher; it breaks down the bodily systems that would help them to be physically and emotionally strong.

3. Instill the Four *S*'s in Your Children

As you set out to foster secure attachment in your children, says Dan Siegel, MD, it can help to remember the basic S's of attachment. Let your child be *seen*, be *safe*, be *soothed*, and feel *secure*.

Seen. Helping our kids to feel seen means perceiving who they are deeply, empathetically. You sense your child's mind beneath her behavior, offer your understanding, and reflect back to her the innate goodness that you see in her. When your child feels as if you see her for who she really is, that you hear and listen to what she thinks and how she feels, that allows her to develop a stronger, more secure attachment. It leads to resilience.

Safe. Avoid actions, reactions, and responses that frighten or hurt your children.

Soothed. Help your children to deal with their difficult emotions and fears. When they encounter fearful or stressful situations, be there for them, with open arms. You are their safe harbor.

Secure. Help your children to develop an internalized sense of well-being by making sure that they know they are safe in the world.

4. Look into Your Child's Eyes

The way in which infants gaze into the eyes of a parent or caregiver is a safety-seeking reflex; it orients them, tells them that they are safe. Eye gaze also matters a lot in helping to ease the impact of adversity and trauma.

One way that we can be a calming, soothing influence is to use what Stephen W. Porges, PhD, professor of psychiatry at the University of North Carolina, Chapel Hill, calls "social engagement behaviors"— including looking into our child's eyes with a deep sense of connectedness. This stimulates the vagus nerve, a critical neural circuit that communicates with the brain, heart, and face, helping to regulate our heart rate, breath, and facial expressions. When we increase the activity of our child's vagus nerve, it has a calming influence on the heart and lungs, and calms the body's hypothalamus-pituitary-adrenal stress axis, turning off the stress response.

If your child is facing a stressful challenge, you can help him or her with a remarkably simple action: stop whatever you're doing, orient yourself so that you are looking deeply into your child's eyes, use your facial muscles to offer a kindhearted, loving gaze—and speak with a soothing tone of voice. You might say, "Let me put what I'm doing down, so that I can give you my full attention." Or, "I really want to hear this."

Just this one, very simple step of gazing eye-to-eye with your child helps him or her to shift out of a fear state and feel seen and secure, all at the same time. That's a lot of healing power in the kind, soothing eye-to-eye parental gaze of love.

When the prefrontal cortex functions with the sense that we are safe and secure in the world, we seek eye contact with other people. We seek connection with them, we want to engage, and we do this by looking into their eyes.

When you make sure to gaze into your children's eyes, you see them for who they really are. You let them see that you witness their innate goodness. You help to establish their sense of safety and secure attachment, without a word.

5. If You Lose It, Apologize—Right Away

If you screw up, you have to make a repair, Dan Siegel, MD, says. Once you've taken a moment to collect yourself, take a breath and come back to center; you can serve your child best by apologizing right away. Siegel suggests saying something along the lines of, "I flipped my lid, and you must have been scared, and I'm sorry." Or, "I lost it and I scared you and I wish I hadn't done that; I'm sorry." When you are able to step in and admit that you were wrong, your child's fear center in the brain—the ever-alert amygdala—stops lighting up. It just calms down.

Recent science on memory and adversity confirms that the quicker we step in, apologize, and make a repair, the less likely it is that an unhappy or frightening memory will stick.

If you are so upset that you can't trust yourself to say the right thing to your child, wait at least ninety seconds. According to Dan Siegel, "After ninety seconds an emotion will arise and fall like a wave on the shore." It takes only ninety seconds to shift out of a mood state, including anger. If you need to, give yourself ninety seconds—about fifteen deep in-and-out breaths—before saying what you need to say to apologize to and soothe your child, so that you can return to a sense of equilibrium and help them feel safe and secure.

Apologizing and admitting that your behavior fell short of the kind of good parenting you're aiming for doesn't diminish you in your children's eyes. Instead, you gain credibility and establish trust. You can even use this as a starting point for an entirely new conversation, perhaps telling your child, "Hey, this is what has been happening, this is why I reacted this way, and I'm sorry. What I said and did was wrong, and I want to do better."

Think of Georgia, and how hard it was for her that her father never apologized after his sudden rages. Or of Mary, whose dad never said, "I'm sorry" for his drunken, sexist behavior. Screwing up is one thing. Being a scary parent and not apologizing doubles the damage.

Bernie Siegel says that "the biggest thing is to say, 'I'm sorry,' so that kids know that they are not to blame for causing whatever problem is at hand."

6. Validate and Normalize All of Your Child's Emotions

Even if you haven't behaved in an ideal manner, once you've owned your mistake, don't obsess about it, Dan Siegel, MD, advises. When you get caught up in your own saga, you aren't really helping your child. Move on to validating and normalizing all of your child's feelings. Don't brush her feelings under the rug or sugarcoat them. Let her be upset, even if she is angry with you. You might say, "I hear you." "That is very frustrating." "That sounds hard."

If your child shares difficult feelings with you, rather than comment or judge, simply say, "Say some more about that?" Or reflect their words back to them: "Let me see if I've got this right so far . . ." Or, "You feel _____ about _____."

Soothing doesn't mean you don't also impose limits. You can send two messages at once, simultaneously accepting all the emotions your child is feeling while still setting limits on his behavior. This allows kids to feel heard but also to know they need to be accountable for their actions. They can't come home late, throw things when angry, scream at you, or not let you know where they are when you ask them to check in.

If you lose it in response to something that your child has done that breaks rules you've clearly established, simply step back, admit that you regret your behavior, apologize, hug, and also make sure he or she understands what behavior prompted your response. You might say, for example, "This must be upsetting. It is hard not to get your way. Our rule, as you know, is that you can't stay out past your curfew, and here are the consequences for that." You can apologize and still stand your ground.

7. Amplify the Good Feelings

We are evolutionarily primed toward worry. Our ancestors were anxious and worried enough to look out vigilantly for predators or other attackers. They passed that genetic proclivity for anxiety on to us. We are a worried species, because worry helped us to survive.

But we need to help our children and ourselves balance the stressful moments, interactions, and even adverse experiences with a sense of wonder and goodness. We need to help our kids look for and take in what's good.

For instance, once you've soothed your toddler after she tells you that someone called her a derogatory name on the playground, you might go on to say, "Wow, you really dealt with that well. That had to be scary and you did just the right thing by coming to tell me."

Or, if you pick up your son from preschool and he is crying because he missed you, you might say, after soothing him, "We are together now, and isn't it nice?" Look for general moments in the day to highlight as positive experiences, paying attention to the good things.

According to neuropsychologist Rick Hanson, PhD, "Since our brain is so primed to take in the negative, it's also important to recognize beneficial experiences in everyday life, and then help turn them into inner strengths such as gratitude, compassion, resilience, and self-worth. When we sustain attention to positive experiences, we help them to be encoded in the brain."

Through using the neural machinery of memory in clever ways, Hanson says, you can defeat the negativity bias of the brain and gain "greater self-confidence, better mood, and a gradual healing of upsetting, even traumatic, experiences."

Researcher John Gottman, MD, PhD, has shown that in any relationship, it typically takes five good interactions to make up for a single bad one. And that's because our painful experiences are a great deal more memorable than pleasurable ones.

As Hanson has put it, "The brain is like Velcro for negative experiences, but Teflon for positive ones." So we need to deliberately "take in the good. When you help your kids do this, over time, the emotional residues of good experiences brighten their worldview." You start to level the playing field, helping them to fire and wire up new, positive neural structures, so that they can develop a brain that is better able to put challenges in perspective. And that, says Hanson, helps children to become more resilient, confident, and happy.

He suggests that we "look for good facts, and turn them into good experiences." You might see a goldfinch or a woodpecker in the garden, or a fish in a pond, a rabbit hopping by, a pretty sunset—just stop and take a moment to stand with your child and talk about the beauty of the moment, the colors you see, the sounds you hear, how pleasant the moment is. Or, says Hanson, you might discuss "how much the two of you are enjoying the taste of a piece of chocolate or a song you love on the radio.

"Savor that moment for ten, twenty, or thirty seconds, to increase its encoding in the brain," says Hanson. "The longer that something is held in awareness and the more emotionally stimulating it is, the more that neurons fire and wire together and the stronger the trace in memory."

You can also do this just before your child is falling asleep—review all the happy or joyful small moments in the day. You might even ask your child to sense the good experience sinking into her—like a warm glow spreading through her chest, or, suggests Hanson, "to imagine a jewel going into the treasure chest of her heart."

Experts recommend that you amplify the good in your child as well. If your son is making a noted effort to complete a tough homework assignment, you might comment, "You sure are persistent." If he holds the door for a person in a wheelchair, "You are so thoughtful!" If your daughter completes a dreaded chore, "You are really responsible." Rather than evaluate her ("You are so smart!" "You're super at that!"), emphasize and name the positive character traits your child exhibits (ingenuity, caring, effort, follow-through, courage, love) out loud, to let her know that you see the good in her.

Meanwhile, as a parent, take in the good *you* notice—people being nice to you in the grocery store, the smell of your child's hair, getting something done at work, finishing the dishes, holding your temper when you're tired, feeling your natural good-heartedness.

8. Stop, Look, Go

Brother David Steindl-Rast, a monk and interfaith scholar, teaches a very simple method to help us to take in the good and be grateful for it. It's so simple, he says, that it's actually what we were taught as children when we learned to cross the street. "*Stop. Look. Go.* That's all it takes," he says. "But how often do we stop? We rush through life. We don't stop. We miss the opportunity because we don't stop." Which means we "have to build stop signs into our lives."

Wherever you are, he says, the more you stop and look, and take in the beauty you see, or the sound of the birds singing, or the clouds crossing the sky, or the feel of someone in your arms—before you go on to what you were about to do next—the more gratitude you feel. And when you feel grateful, you feel a deeper sense of happiness and joy—the ultimate antidote to inflammatory stress.

By helping your kids, and yourself, to actively "stop and look" for beauty in our world, for signs of how others care for you, or good qualities within you, by soaking in those good feelings before you "go" on to the next thing, you're helping to counter the impact of childhood CUTS.

9. Give a Name to Difficult Emotions

Matthew Lieberman, PhD, professor of psychology at the University of California, Los Angeles, has found that when you name your emotions, you activate areas of the brain that help you to react less. If you help your children to name what's happening inside them—to say the words, "I'm feeling angry and afraid right now"—their alarm-center response in their brains turns down significantly. The more you help your children to exercise this part of the brain that names feelings, the less stressed they will be, even when stressful things are happening to them.

Dan Siegel, MD, puts it simply: "Name it to tame it."

If your child can't name what's happening, try offering him or her options. "Are you feeling mad, or sad, or afraid?" You might even consider writing down this question and offering multiple-choice answers. Or you might try opening the conversation by imagining how they are feeling: "What happened was really scary. Are you feeling scared?" Help your children learn to name their emotions before they are overtaken by them.

Remind your children that the problem is not their feeling of anxiety, fear, or anger; the problem is how they react when they feel overwhelmed. By helping your children to name all the difficult feelings, you help to keep them from acting out, feeling overwhelmed, or shutting down.

10. The Incredible Power of the Twenty-Second Hug

When children feel safe in engaging, interacting, and bonding with you, they move toward you, allowing you to help them to regulate their emotional distress. This is the essence of secure attachment. One way you can enhance this process is through giving your kids a twenty-second full-body hug. It sounds so simple, and yet we're often moving so fast that our hugs are short and rushed.

When you hold your child and hug for twenty seconds, the sense of touch and warmth releases the "bonding hormone," oxytocin. Oxytocin calms down the amygdala, and, recent studies show, even helps to increase production of GABA, which is essential to brain function and helps to promote a sense of calm.

11. Make "What's Happening" a Safe and Open Conversation

One of the reasons that childhood adversity is so damaging is not only that it's happening, but that it often happens in secret. Kids code secrets as being bad. If the adversity they face is being kept secret and no one is talking about it, something must be wrong. But rather than assume something is wrong with their situation, kids interpret secrets to mean they themselves must be bad, stupid, or wrong. They feel at fault, as if by being less than perfect they somehow brought on a situation.

Acknowledge what's happening. Bring the conversation out into the open. This can be pivotal for a child, when done supportively and safely.

Laura's mother's sister, to whom she'd always been close, helped her to realize she wasn't alone with the secret of her mother's cruelty. "Looking back, I think my aunt saved my life," she says. "One day when

I was fourteen, she came and sat on my bed and said, 'It's not you, okay? It's her problem—I want you to know that what's happening, it's *not you*.' It doesn't sound like much, but all those years, alone with my mom's constant critiques, I thought there had to be something so wrong with me. Why else would my mom always be criticizing me? I didn't hear other moms talking to their kids that way. That ten-second conversation with my aunt gave me this glimmer of hope that maybe it wasn't all me; maybe I wasn't so despicable, maybe I wasn't grossly un-lovable. That was the dawning of my awareness that maybe something was wrong with my mom. I sometimes wonder, if my aunt hadn't sat on the side of my bed and said those eighteen words, would I have made it through my teenage years? Would I still be here?"

When you bring forth the truth of what's happening, you give kids the opportunity to go from feeling utterly alone, asking themselves, "What is wrong with me that this is happening?" and assuming they are inherently bad and deserve what's occurring, to asking themselves far healthier questions: "What is wrong with the person who is doing this to me?" "What is wrong with this situation?"

When you speak the truth, you help kids to make this critical, es-sential leap that they are not the problem; they are not unworthy or un-lovable. Once you help them to make that leap, they have a far greater possibility of healing.

Cindy's oldest son is sixteen now. She says, "We can talk about hard things." She has learned to tell her son "if I am facing a lot of emotions that are based on something old, something from my childhood. I ac-knowledge that it is there, let him know I'm handling it, and move on." As a child, Cindy had a strong sense that there was always the prover-bial elephant in the room, and that so much went unacknowledged. Her father was obviously treating people abusively and no one ever called him on it and said, "Hey, this is not okay, what is he doing? Are those kids okay?"

Now, when Cindy is struggling, "when I feel that the past is hugely impacting me or how I parent in the present, I give my kids the biggest gift I have to give them: I let them know, 'Hey, here is what is happening,' and then we can have a conversation that is open and safe. I believe one of the best things I can do for my kids is to share my own experiences, name the challenges I've faced, and offer what I've learned. I'm far from a perfect parent; sometimes my anxiety from the past catches up with me. But by letting my kids know that, they know that it is not their fault, this is *my* stuff. Why would I not give them that simple gift?"

12. Reframe Stories of Intergenerational Trauma

Once you understand that your adversity was inherited from preceding generations' adversity, you can tell a larger narrative that encompasses the story of your parents, grandparents, yourself, and your children.

Kendall has been able to have compassion for her dad, when she considers how it must have hurt him to have had his mother commit suicide when he was a boy, and to have his family try to keep it a secret. "Certainly that played a role in his becoming an alcoholic." It also "helps me to understand why he never stood up for me, even when my mother was abusive. He needed to believe that she was perfect, invincible, given that his own mom's imperfections were, to him, synonymous with death and the loss of everything he'd known." Kendall has developed compassion for her mother, too. "I realize now that it couldn't have been easy for her to live with my father's depression and alcoholism. She had perfected a neurotic way of coping: when things upset her or made her uncomfortable, she insisted everything was fine. She pretended my father was fine, she pretended that I was fine. And she'd learned that dysfunctional coping mechanism from her own upbringing."

Knowing all this doesn't change what happened, Kendall says, "but it has helped me to understand that this didn't begin with me. And understanding this has made me even more determined that this toxic intergenerational legacy will end."

Georgia feels similarly. She says, "My family's multigenerational pattern gives me insight, it makes it less personal, less about me. My grandmother was abandoned as a baby. She was a very injured person. So she was very abusive to my mother. My mother was deeply injured, and so she became like her mother. A similar pattern played itself out on my father's side. These patterns were well in effect before I came along."

John has found it easier to reach out to his father with the recognition that "my father's home life growing up was even more difficult than mine," he says. "His mother was a single mom at eighteen, and he never knew who his father was. He never really had anyone who was there for him. And so he didn't grow up with much emotional intelligence."

Understanding how adversity and trauma are inherited helps you to reframe your children's story into a story that is less based on your own past and, therefore, less personal. By making sense of the web of family stories, you can recognize how your own experience has been authored by others before you were even born. You can see how to break those emotional shackles, and set out to avoid carrying remnants of your parents' injury into your children's future.

13. A Child Needs a Reliable Adult or Mentor

The best way to prevent or remediate toxic stress, says Jack Shonkoff, MD, is "having adults who are there to help children get through, to help them feel a sense of safety, feel a sense of protection, and most important, to begin to build their own capacities to be able to deal and cope with stress." Often, children are in trouble because they feel no sense of buffering and protection around them. They lack "consistent, protective, reliable, supportive relationships with caring adults to help them get through and learn to deal with adversity."

What kids need most when there is a sense of threat, and they are caught up in an ongoing stress response, is to know that there is someone they can count on. Adversity is colored by the context in which events happen. And that context has everything to do with whether there are adults to help a child through.

According to Dan Siegel, MD, reliable adult relationships are one of the most important factors in establishing childhood resiliency. And this includes having adults outside of the family to whom a child can turn, especially during the tumult of adolescence. Throughout human history, Siegel points out, "We stayed together as communities, with adolescents exploring and establishing independence while maintaining a range of important and instructive interactions with their adult elders." Those strands of connectedness between generations "are being stretched thin in today's world. We don't really have that in our culture. But kids need to have other nonparental adults around, whether they are teachers, mentors, or coaches."

When children are still young, a mentor, a safe reliable adult, is a "place" where they can go so that they know they are not alone, a safe haven. To have one wise voice offering them sound advice, comfort, faith in themselves and who they are can make all the difference.

Mentoring groups who work with at-risk youth and in underserved populations use a rubric that includes forty developmental assets for adolescents, one of which is "other adult relationships." Mentoring groups suggest that young people receive support from three or more nonparent adults. Those relationships don't take the place of developing a secure attachment with a primary caregiver, but having other safe, reliable adults in their lives can help kids to believe in themselves, in their own goodness.

Bernie Siegel, MD, tells the story of helping to take care of a teenager who faced a great deal of early adversity and who was often suicidal. One day, this young girl came in to see him and said, "You're my CD." Siegel asked her what she meant. "She told me, 'You're my Chosen Dad.' That is the impact we can have on a young person who is suffering when we let kids know that they are safe with us, and that we love them."

In the course of doing interviews for this book, many individuals said that there was one person in their life who acted as a mentor, who stepped in to provide a safe environment—what we might think of as an emotional benefactor. And having that one, safe reliable adult helped them get through, until they grew up and were able to turn their experiences into grist for deeper understanding and growth.

Even in the midst of Mary's erratic home life, she had her friend Andrea's mom, who always had a spare bed for her, who taught her how to bake. "Andrea's mom was familiar with my dad's drinking and how he spanked us; she knew that he'd get loud and angry, and that there were these terrible pictures on the walls, but she still loved me," Mary says. "Andrea wasn't allowed to come to my house; I was always welcome at their house, no matter what time or day it was."

Cindy tells a similar story. "We had neighbors down the street who were so good to me. They could that see things had fallen apart in my house, and they told me that I should consider their invitation to come over 'an open-door policy.' I was over there every day, for years. I'd even go on vacation with them. Looking back, I realize that their family, and the mom especially, played an enormous role in helping me to get through my childhood. She never turned me away."

Kendall talks about her older female friend who had watched how hard it had been for Kendall growing up, and who helped Kendall make sense of her past, encouraging her to seek therapy.

For others it might be a special family member, an aunt or a grandparent. For John, it was his mother's mother. "She was just such a huge influence in my life," he says. She always let me know that she loved me unconditionally. She was the opposite of my father. Every chance she had she would tell me, 'I love you.' I loved her with my whole heart. We would walk her dog and the moon would be out and she'd just hold my hand and talk to the moon, 'Oh, hello, moon,' she'd say. She helped me to see the beauty in the world through her eyes. I think she might have saved me. Now, when I walk outside to take out the trash and see the moon up in the sky, I think of her. I think of how her love was the one great thing in my childhood."

Kat feels her life might have been saved by the love of her grandmother, or G-Ma, and the few years she spent living with her at the end of high school. "It was just the two of us," she recalls. "She never lost patience with me, no matter how surly or quiet or defiant I was. She drove me everywhere I needed to go. She made me a bagged lunch every day and wrote my name on it with a big, black marker. When I was sick, she dropped everything to stay home with me and take care of me. She made me homemade chicken soup. I started to call her my G-Ma. That one relationship, her love, made an enormous difference for me—though I didn't understand that at the time." Kat recalls how, when she began her first teaching job, her G-Ma sent her a card on which she'd written, *Kat, Your mom would have been so proud of you.* Her grandmother had underlined each word three times. "It had been a long time since anyone had acknowledged that I'd missed having my mom," Kat says. "It felt like the first time in my life that anyone had said they were proud of anything I'd done."

Shortly after that, her grandmother died.

"I don't think I would have been able to find that small part of me inside that felt that maybe I deserved to heal, if I hadn't had a brief period when I lived with my grandmother, if she hadn't been there to love me," Kat says.

14. Bring Mindfulness into Schools

During the school year nearly half of a child's waking hours are spent at school, which can be a high-stress climate with a great deal of pressure to compete and achieve. Bullying and social exclusion can add to the stress.

American teenagers cite their stress level as being a six on a scale of ten during the school year. In summer, their stress levels drop strikingly. So we have to ask ourselves whether it makes sense to have so much of an American teen's day taken up with high-stakes performance-based endeavors—studying, tests, exams, AP tests, SATs, ACTs.

In 2014, hundreds of educators gathered in Washington, DC, for the Mindfulness in Education Conference and to explore how to bring compassion and mindfulness into our schools. One of the conference leaders, Jack Kornfield, PhD, noted that teachers and educators are beginning to understand that "when you are trying to teach a child and their parents are in the midst of a divorce, how are they supposed to come and be quiet at their desk and learn how to write an essay?"

We need to look at kids' home and school stress levels, and give them the skills to manage or decrease their stress.

Recent studies show that learning mindfulness and meditation improve mental health, grades, and decrease stress in high school students. One study found that students who take a ten-minute lesson in mindfulness meditation stay less stressed during high-stakes math exams, scoring on average five points higher in math than other students. Individuals trained in meditation perform significantly better on standardized tests that require focused attention, and adolescent boys who take four forty-minute classes and practice with a CD for eight or more minutes a day experience a greater feeling of well-being.

Another study found that adolescents who took a course on mindfulness had less depression and lower stress levels—and the more they practiced mindfulness, the less stressed they felt and the greater well-being they experienced, even three months after the study. Christina Bethell, PhD, professor at Johns Hopkins Bloomberg School of Public Health, found that children with two or more ACEs who had developed some aspects of resilience—such as the ability to stay calm and in control when faced with a challenge—were over one and a half times more likely to be engaged with their classwork compared to similar children with two or more ACEs who had not learned resilience.

Meanwhile, schools are starting to pay attention to the fact that students may be dealing with trauma at home, in their neighborhoods, and even at their schools. In one school in the state of Washington, administrators implemented trauma-informed practices to help support kids who may be facing adversity at home. Their goal was to change their discipline system from "a blame-shame-punishment approach" to one of taking care of kids—and teachers—so that kids can learn. They found that in a kindergarten-to-fifth-grade school setting of 275 students in the more caring environment, suspensions plummeted by 89 percent and kids were expelled less frequently. According to Jane Stevens, founder and editor of ACEsTooHigh.com, a news site, and ACEsConnection, a social network whose members are implementing practices based on ACE research, "Trauma-sensitive schools are better schools." Hundreds of schools are taking up this trauma-based approach, but, says Stevens, "we need to take this to a national level to have broad impact."

This also means we need to help train teachers to be mindful, too. Robert Whitaker MD, a pediatrician and professor of pediatrics and public health at Temple University, has been looking at how mindfulness protects people from the physical and mental health effects of Adverse Childhood Experiences. Working with more than two thousand teachers and staff in Head Start programs, he found that many of these individuals had suffered from ACEs, but those who practiced mindfulness reported more positive mental and physical health outcomes no matter how many ACEs they'd experienced.

When teachers stay mindful and calm, even when kids show behavioral or other problems, they are better able to create a safe environment for their students. Whitaker says, "The presence or connection with other adults who can help make sense of the meaning of one's life in the context of suffering helps a child become resilient." It's essential to have "a compassionate response from a person with whom the child feels safe."

"How we help our talented teachers to reduce their stress levels matters, too," says Stevens.

As parents, caregivers, and educators, we can ask parent-teacher associations and schools to bring in mindfulness programs for our children and to emphasize learning how to manage stressful feelings as part of a well-rounded education for success.

In Conclusion

Childhood adversity can tear you down but it can also be your single greatest impetus for growth. It takes tremendous courage and inner strength to transform the trauma of childhood adversity into a journey toward post-traumatic growth. But when you do reorient yourself, you open to the possibility of healing.

It's important to walk a fine line between embracing the complexity of ACE science, and assuming it means you will never have the chance for a happy, fulfilling and contented life.

Writer Andrew Solomon, author *The Noonday Demon: An Atlas of Depression* as well as *Far from the Tree: Parents, Children, and the Search for Identity*, talks about having endured the torment of bullying as a child for being "different"—he would ultimately realize those differences were all connected to his being gay. "Those early experiences can be very powerful and very determinative; you end up developing an image of yourself, an image of what your strengths are, an image of your weaknesses, an image of the ways in which the world is going to limit you."

However, says Solomon, "You need to take the traumas and make them part of who you've come to be," folding "the worst events of your life into a narrative of triumph, evincing a better self in response to things that hurt."

"We cannot bear a pointless torment," Solomon says, "but we can endure great pain if we believe that it's purposeful." Indeed, it is "our misfortunes that drive our search for meaning."

The recognition that you have lived through hard times also drives you to develop deeper empathy, seek more intimacy, value life's sweeter moments, and treasure your connectedness to others and to the world at large. This is the hard-won benefit of having known suffering.

Researchers have found that in the last decades of life, between the ages of sixty-five and eighty-four, those who never suffered from childhood adversity have *greater* levels of inflammatory hormones than do those who faced childhood adversity. Perhaps over time, as we begin to make meaning of our experiences, incorporate our past into our complex identity, and accept how it has shaped who we are now, we ultimately gain some deeper sense of self and self-acceptance.

People who met up with adversity in the past have "an elevated capacity for savoring," say researchers, who also concluded that "the worst experiences in life may come with an eventual upside, by promoting the ability to appreciate life's small pleasures."

Ultimately, when you embrace the process of healing despite your Adverse Childhood Experiences, you don't just become who you might have been if you hadn't encountered so much childhood suffering in the first place. You gain something better: the hard-earned gift of life wisdom, which you bring forward into every arena of your life.

New Medical Horizons

It has been said that if child abuse and neglect were to disappear today, the *Diagnostic and Statistical Manual* would shrink to the size of a pamphlet in two generations, and the prisons would empty.

Or, as Bernie Siegel, MD, puts it, quite simply, after half a century of practicing medicine, "I have become convinced that our number-one public health problem is our childhood."

The biological Theory of Everything—that Adverse Childhood Experiences shape who we are and who we become, physically, neurologically, emotionally—has been mind-bogglingly slow to change "how we 'do medicine,'" says Vincent Felitti, MD. "Very few internists or medical schools are interested in embracing the added responsibility that this understanding imposes on them."

This is particularly dumbfounding given that physicians need all the help they can get "to uncover the root causes of chronic, intractable illness, pain, and distress," says Felitti. Understanding ACE research allows us a new avenue in an area where medicine has largely failed: helping patients who have been suffering from decades of chronic illness with little hope.

"As physicians," says Felitti, "we know that there are really only three sources of diagnostic information: patient history, physical examination, and laboratory testing. While patients overwhelmingly assume that diagnosis derives from lab tests, very experienced physicians will tell you that 75 to 80 percent of the time diagnosis derives from the patient history." Moreover, Felitti adds, "The incorporation of trauma-oriented questions, which we have now used with 440,000 adult patients over an eight-year period, can help us to know in advance where we need to go and where we don't need to go with a patient."

There is no question, Felitti says, "that it is easier to respond to the symptoms that a patient is presenting in the moment, than it is to understand why that problem exists in the first place, especially if the problem is chronic. But when physicians seek to understand people's lives as well as their biomedical bodies and symptoms, we create a new possibility for patients to find wellness."

Indeed, there appears to be a direct health benefit for adult patients when they are helped to recognize and discuss the potential link between their childhood experiences and adult health problems. In one recent study of 125,000 patients, Felitti found that those who took the ACE Study questionnaire as part of their medical history and who discussed their ACE Scores with their doctors had a 35 percent reduction in their doctor visits and an 11 percent reduction in emergency room visits over the course of the following year. This was especially true for adult patients with chronic illness, whose illnesses were particularly difficult to treat.

But as health-care dollars have become stretched, physicians are spending less time interacting one-on-one with patients in their exam rooms; the average physician schedules patients back to back at fifteen-minute intervals. By *Asking, Listening,* and *Accepting,* however, physicians are able "to provide great relief to our patients," says Felitti. In a clinical setting, a clinician might say, "I see that on the questionnaire [your father was an alcoholic/you were sexually assaulted/your mother had bipolar disorder/your brother committed suicide/you were frequently made fun of as a kid]. Can you tell me how that has affected you later in life?"

Counter to many physicians' fears that this question might lead to "opening Pandora's Box in the exam room," says Felitti, patients' responses lasted only a few brief minutes. But those few moments helped physicians obtain a depth and breadth of patient information that had a "profound and beneficial impact on patient care," helping their patients change their healing trajectory toward well-being.

But seeing that connection takes a little time. It means asking a patient to fill out the simple Adverse Childhood Experiences questionnaire to screen them for ACEs as part of an initial written intake and verbally asking them about their childhood during an exam. It requires reading that patient's history for insight into sources of both physical and emotional pain. It might mean actually sitting down with a patient—which, studies show, physicians do only 9 percent of the time—and perhaps even giving them a gesture of comfort such as shaking their hand or putting a hand on their shoulder. It will certainly mean offering them appropriate steps toward healing in addition to the best that traditional medicine has to offer.

With the ACE research now available, we might hope that physicians will begin to see patients as a holistic sum of their experiences and embrace the understanding that a stressor from long ago can be a health-risk time bomb that has exploded. Such a medical paradigm, which sees Adverse Childhood Experiences as one of many key factors that can play a role in disease, could save many patients years in the healing process.

The cost of not intervening is far greater—not only in the loss of human health and well-being but also in health-care dollars. According to the Centers for Disease Control and Prevention, the total lifetime cost of child maltreatment in the United States is $124 billion each year. The lifetime health-care cost for each individual who experiences childhood maltreatment is estimated to be $210,012—which is comparable to other costly health conditions, such as having a stroke, which has a lifetime estimated cost of $159,846 per person, or type 2 diabetes, which is estimated to cost between $181,000 and $253,000.

Further hindering change is the fact that physical adult medicine and psychological medicine remain in separate silos. Utilizing ACE research in how we "do medicine" requires breaking down these long-standing divisions in health care between what is "physical" and what is "mental" or "emotional." And that is hard to do. Physicians have been well trained to deal with only what they can touch with their hands, see with their eyes, or view with microscopes or scans.

However, now that we have scientific evidence that the brain is genetically modified by childhood experience, we can no longer draw that line in the sand. Hundreds of studies have shown that childhood adversity hurts our mental and physical health, putting us at greater risk for learning disorders, cardiovascular disease, autoimmune disease, depression, obesity, suicide, substance abuse, failed relationships, violence, poor parenting, and early death.

Dr. Jeffrey Brenner, a 2013 MacArthur Foundation genius award winner, recently stated, "ACE Scores should become a vital sign, as important as height, weight, and blood pressure. There was a time when physicians were reluctant to ask about and address smoking, unsafe sexual activity, and obesity. The taboos and discomfort about discussing childhood traumas with patients need to be lifted as well."

Hopeful Frontiers in Pediatric Medicine

Meanwhile, there is hope closer at hand. Change is afoot in pediatric medicine and education. Jack Shonkoff, MD, the director of Harvard's Center on the Developing Child, believes that the new science on toxic stress in childhood will inspire subspecialists in medicine to share data and treatment systems. "It's one science," Shonkoff emphasizes in a recent radio interview. "It's as much about health as it is about education. It's as much about pediatrics as it is about gerontology." With the scientific evidence at hand, he says, "Now you have both a science-based imperative and a moral responsibility to say, 'We can't allow this to go by.' We must respond urgently to this, as we have to other public health threats."

In June 2014, the Academy of American Pediatrics, or AAP, convened a symposium on the long-term dangers of childhood toxic stress, urging pediatricians, policy makers, and federal agencies to develop a stronger national response. To help further those efforts, the AAP has recently launched a new Center on Healthy, Resilient Children, which will promote education for pediatricians and other clinicians on protecting the brain during development, provide tools to help pediatricians screen families for traumatic stress, and connect parents with appropriate resources.

Robert W. Block, MD, past president of AAP, and head of the Center on Healthy, Resilient Children, says "Pediatric medicine now recognizes the real and significant effects when children grow up with toxic and persistent stress."

The battle to help intervene in the lives of children facing adversity and trauma has, however, only just begun. According to Robin Karr-Morse, "We are a nation of idiots about infancy. We are the only postindustrial First World nation that hasn't signed the U.N. Rights of the Child. We have a huge black eye in our nation regarding our rate of child abuse and neglect." Adding to the problem is the fact that, "our child care system in this country is still deplorable. It is simply not keeping up with the need. We're leaving a lot of children behind."

So far, the greatest changes are happening, slowly, in pediatrics, social services, the juvenile justice system, and K–12 educational settings that serve at-risk students. Living in poverty and violence can add to an accumulation of stress that blunts individuals' learning potential, and derails their emotional and physical health, for life. This gives us a new framework to rethink our schools and how schools can become more trauma-sensitive to students.

Adverse Childhood Experiences research also should prompt new questions about military service and who should serve, potentially using ACE questionnaires as a screening tool to help determine who might be more prone to long-term PTSD—as well as to help encourage those returning from combat to seek treatment to lessen their trauma. ACE research also shows a new way to help understand and treat addiction by seeing it as self-medicating—an unsuccessful attempt to lessen the pain created by adversity.

In some cities, counties, and states, people from different sectors such as health care, business, child welfare, and schools are coming together to make their communities trauma-informed and resilient. Nearly thirty states, including Washington State, Iowa, Maine, and Vermont, have already begun collecting Adverse Childhood Experiences data in order to better develop state public health programs that address child and family problems, including child abuse, domestic violence, and substance abuse.

"Communities are working together to change organizations and systems to replace blame-shame-punishment rules and policies with understanding-nurturing-solutions and approaches," says Jane Stevens, founder of the news site ACEsConnection.com and the social network ACEsTooHigh.com. "Although much of the reason for doing this is economic—it can save a city hundreds of millions of dollars in reduced costs for health care and social services—it also helps people and their communities to become healthier and happier places to live."

Meanwhile, real people are hurting.

—

I encourage you to go take a look at the adult you see in the mirror, and try to see, in your eyes, the child you once were. Pay attention to his or her story. Think back to the many strategies and modalities now available to help you come back to who it is you really are—and become even better, wiser, stronger for the journey. And promise that child you once were that you will take him or her on a quest to heal.

LET'S CONTINUE THE CONVERSATION ABOUT ADVERSE CHILDHOOD EXPERIENCES

In order to help further our conversation, connect us, and help you to find and share resources and stories of hope, I invite you to join me on my community forums. You can do this in one of three ways:

- Join my community discussion on my Facebook page at https://www.facebook.com/donnajacksonnakazawaauthor.
- Join my CHILDHOOD INTERRUPTED blog at www.donnajacksonnakazawa.com.
- Be part of my CHILDHOOD DISRUPTED group forum on AcesConnection.com, at http://www.acesconnection.com/g/childhood-disrupted, where I'm moderating a CHILDHOOD DISRUPTED discussion group. All are invited.

I'll look forward to hearing from you. Let's work together by sharing stories about how to find a healing path—so that you can finally live the life you deserve.

ACKNOWLEDGMENTS

Being grateful for the good in one's life is one of many ways to enhance well-being, and I'm glad to have a chance to express my appreciation here to the many people who helped make this book possible.

My reporting benefited from the generosity and wisdom of many scholars, scientists, and researchers, but I am especially grateful to Vincent J. Felitti, MD, for his kindness, generosity, and patience during our many conversations and communications. As the "scientific fathers" of Adverse Childhood Experiences research, Felitti and Robert Anda, MD, have created a life-changing paradigm for better understanding human suffering and healing. I am grateful to them for allowing me to delve into their findings.

The generosity of spirit shown by the following leading experts and thinkers in the fields of neuroscience, neurobiology, and immunology provided great help, and none of them should underestimate how helpful they have been: Margaret McCarthy, PhD, professor of neuroscience at the University of Maryland School of Medicine, welcomed me to shadow her in her lab, and served as an unflagging scientific advisor to whom I turned when I had questions large and small. De-Lisa Fairweather, PhD, associate professor of toxicology at the Johns Hopkins Bloomberg School of Public Health and the Mayo Clinic, generously helped me understand her important work on women and Adverse Childhood Experiences, and how these intersect with female immunology. Dan Siegel, MD, child neuropsychiatrist and clinical professor at the University of California, Los Angeles (UCLA); neuropsychiatrist Ryan Herringa, MD, PhD, assistant professor of child and adolescent psychiatry at the University of Wisconsin; and Ruth Lanius, MD, PhD, neuroscientist and professor of psychiatry and director of the post-traumatic stress disorder (PTSD) research unit at the University of Western Ontario in Canada, generously provided time and insights so that I might better understand how Adverse Childhood Experiences affect the developing brain, our interpersonal biology, and early development.

I am grateful to the following individuals for conversations that shaped my understanding of their work and findings: Bernie Siegel, MD; Francine Shapiro, PhD, senior research fellow at the Mental Research Institute in Palo Alto, California; Mark D. Seery, PhD, associate professor of psychology at the University at Buffalo; Kerry Ressler, MD, PhD, professor of psychiatry and behavioral sciences at Emory's department of psychiatry and behavioral sciences; and Vicki Abeles, documentarist of *Race to Nowhere*.

I'm indebted to the following scientists, experts, and scholars for email exchanges that provided clarity on their work: neuropsychologist Rick Hanson, PhD, Senior Fellow of the Greater Good Science Center; Robin Karr-Morse, family therapist; Seth Pollak, PhD, professor of psychology and director of the Child Emotion Research Laboratory at the University of Wisconsin; Joan Kaufman, PhD, director of the Child and Adolescent Research and Education (CARE) program at Yale School of Medicine; Hilary P. Blumberg, MD, professor of psychiatry and director of the Mood Disorders Research Program at Yale School of Medicine; Robert Whitaker, MD, professor of pediatrics and public health at Temple University; Robert W. Block, MD, past president of AAP, and head of the Center on Healthy, Resilient Children; Bruce S. McEwen, PhD, professor of neuroendocrinology at Rockefeller University; and Stanford University psychologist Kelly

McGonigal, PhD. Thanks also to Jack Kornfield, PhD, Buddhist meditation teacher and psychologist; Tara Brach, PhD, meditation teacher and psychologist; and James Gordon, MD, founder and director of the Center for Mind-Body Medicine in Washington, DC, for allowing me to quote their teachings, and to Al Race, director of Communications and Public Engagement at the Center on the Developing Child at Harvard University, for his help in quoting the work of Jack Shonkoff, MD, director of the Center on the Developing Child at Harvard University.

A special heartfelt thanks to writer Andrew Solomon.

I am likewise indebted to Jane Stevens, journalist and founder of the social network ACEsConnection.com and the news site ACEs TooHigh.com—to whom the field of ACE research owes so much.

This book could not have been written without the intrepid, brave individuals who allowed me to tell their stories of trauma and recovery. I am indebted to every one of you, and I hope this book honors your stories, your healing, and your determination to create meaningful lives regardless of the obstacles encountered.

To my agent and dear friend, Elizabeth Kaplan, your encouragement for my lifelong mission to change the world by bringing light to what causes pain, suffering, and illness, and to help readers understand what creates and affirms healing, has made it possible for me to do this work. Thanks for your faith in me. My gratitude to Leslie Meredith at Atria for seeing the value in this book, and for her careful, mindful edits, as well as to Donna Loffredo for her kindness and good cheer in keeping the process running smoothly. To my friend Lee Kravitz, thank you for making the early chapters of this book a better read.

To my friends in my Advanced Readers Circle, Jen Britton, Leslie Hoffmeister, Sarah Judd, Barbee Whitaker ("Seesta"), thank you for reading early pages, commenting, and making my life better by being in it. Kimberly Minear, a heartfelt thanks for reading, and for your support, and welcome distractions along the way, without which I might not have made it through this rapid production cycle.

Thank you to the Virginia Center for the Creative Arts, for allowing me much-needed time to finish this book.

Finally, and most important, thanks to my husband, Zenji, who helped me get through the sixteen-hour writing days by supporting me in every way possible, with Paleo dinners, endless hugs, patience, and good humor. And to my children, for their perhaps misguided faith that my writing can help make the world a healthier place ("Mom, you can do it!"). My desire for them, and for the next generation, to thrive, is perhaps the greatest driving force behind this book that you now hold in your hands.

NOTES

Introduction

xiv *The ACE Study measured ten types of adversity:* The World Health Organization's "Adverse Childhood Experiences International Questionnaire" examines the link between community violence, peer violence, domestic violence, and later adult health outcomes: http://www.who.int/violence_injury_prevention/violence/activities/adverse_childhood_experiences/en/ (accessed March 29, 2015).

Chapter One: Every Adult Was Once a Child

11 *Felitti came to this realization almost:* Vincent J. Felitti recounts the history of how he came to understand the role of trauma in his patients' health when he began to investigate why patients who were successfully losing weight at his obesity clinic at Kaiser were dropping out of the program. It didn't make sense; the clinic was helping these same patients to accomplish previously unheard of weight losses, something they claimed to want. And yet they were leaving when they started succeeding. In order to understand why, Felitti decided to meet with them one-on-one. He began interviewing them with a time-line approach, asking, "What did you weigh at birth, in kindergarten, in sixth grade, and if you can't recall, were you the fattest kid in class, the thinnest, or regular size?" For some time two nurses in Kaiser's weight program who worked with Felitti had occasionally hinted to him about patients referring to "sexual issues." So Felitti intended to ask patients their age when they first became sexually active. But in one of his interviews he misspoke and asked a woman how much she had weighed when she first became sexually active. She answered, "Forty pounds," and then sobbed the words, "It was with my father." Not knowing what to do or how to respond, Dr. Felitti slowly continued the time line and learned that shortly after being sexually abused, his patient's weight gain began. Ten days later he stumbled across another childhood sexual abuse case, in which an interviewee talked about early abuse, and he began to pursue this issue routinely with all the obesity patients he was seeing. The results were staggering, causing him to initially doubt his findings. "It seemed that every other person I questioned acknowledged a history of childhood sexual abuse," Felitti says. He thought, "This can't be. People would know if this

241

were true. Someone would have told me. Wasn't that what medical school was for?" Over several months Felitti collected 186 such cases in the weight program. When he reviewed his records, it turned out that 55 percent of the patients he interviewed in the obesity program acknowledged a history of sexual assault. He had five colleagues interview the next hundred patients in the obesity program, to make sure he wasn't somehow showing bias. They got the same results. Felitti became convinced that "this relationship between early trauma and obesity was real but that no one wanted to know this," he says. "Most colleagues even felt that such questions couldn't be asked, and told me, 'You can't ask questions like that! Patients will be furious and no one will tell you the truth anyway.'" The Adverse Childhood Experiences Study was born out of these "counterintuitive observations in the obesity program," including "our discovery of the *threat* imposed by major weight loss," says Felitti. In other words, women who have faced trauma may unconsciously want to keep weight on as a defense against sexual advances and abuse, and men who have been abused may unconsciously want to keep weight on as protection (as in "throwing your weight around"). This early history on Felitti's experiences as a physician prior to developing the Adverse Childhood Experiences Survey, both in the text of this book, and here, comes from email exchanges on February 2, 2015 as well as conversations with Vincent J. Felitti, MD, over the past two years.

11 *It became clear to him that for his patients:* V.J. Felitti, K. Jakstis, V. Pepper, et al., "Obesity: Problem, Solution, or Both?," *The Permanente Journal.* 14, no. 1 (Spring 2010), 24–30, 29.

12 *He suggested that Felitti set up:* This early history of events leading up to the development of the Adverse Childhood Experiences Survey comes from an email exchange with Vincent J. Felitti, MD, on February 2, 2015: "I presented my findings at a national obesity conference in Atlanta in 1990, where I was attacked by the audience, but also met Dr. David Williamson from the CDC; this was where the ACE Study began. Seated next to me at a speakers' dinner, David Williamson said, 'Look, if what you're saying is true, it has enormous importance for the nation as well as for the practice of medicine. But no one is going to believe your 286 cases no matter how well you've studied them. What we need is an epidemiologically sound study involving thousands of patients, and from a *general* population, not some unusual subset that you've accumulated in an obesity program.' After a moment's reflection, I told David that I had such a place back in San Diego. Our Health Appraisal Division of Kaiser Permanente's Department of Preventive Medicine was providing unusually comprehensive and standardized medical examination and evaluation to 58,000 adults a year. We discussed how many were 'enough' and concluded that 26,000 would be a workable number. I was then invited to speak at the CDC, and several senior CDC people came out to visit." This early history on Felitti's experiences as a physician prior to developing the Adverse Childhood Experiences Survey, both in the text of this book, and here, comes from email exchanges on February 2, 2015, as well as conversations with Vincent J. Felitti, MD, over the past two years.

13 *After the interviews, each participant:* Robert F. Anda, MD, spent several years trav-

eling back and forth between Atlanta and San Diego, building and assembling the ACE questionnaire, and later running the analysis of the ACE Study findings, with the help of a team he supervised at the CDC. This early history on Anda's development of the ACE questionnaire, survey, and findings comes from a conversation with Robert F. Anda, MD, on April 8, 2015.

14 *And 87 percent of those who answered yes:* V. J. Felitti and R. F. Anda, "The Relationship of Adverse Childhood Experiences to Adult Medical Disease, Psychiatric Disorders, and Sexual Behavior: Implications for Healthcare," in *The Effects of Early Life Trauma on Health and Disease: The Hidden Epidemic,* edited by R. Lanius, E. Vermetten, C. Pain (New York: Cambridge University Press. 2010), 77.

14 *Forty percent had experienced two or more:* Ibid.

14 *Here, says Felitti, "was the missing piece":* For more on Vincent J. Felitti and Robert F. Anda's original ACE Study and findings, see V. J. Felitti and R. F. Anda, "The Lifelong Effects of Adverse Childhood Experiences," in *Child Maltreatment: Sexual Abuse and Psychological Maltreatment,* Vol. 2, edited by D. L. Chadwick, A. P. Giardino, R. Alexander, et al., (St. Louis, MO): STM Learning, 2014), 203–15.

14 *People with an ACE Score of 4 were twice as likely:* S. R. Dube, R. F. Anda, V. J. Felitti, et al., "Growing Up with Parental Alcohol Abuse: Exposure to Childhood Abuse, Neglect, and Household Dysfunction," *Child Abuse and Neglect* 25, no. 12 (December 2001), 1627–40. Also see H. Larkin and J. Records, "Adverse Childhood Experiences: Overview, Response Strategies and Integral Theory Perspective" (2006): 13. This article originally appeared in the *Journal of Integral Theory and Practice* 2, issue no. 3, in a slightly different form; onse.org/img/uploads/file/larkin_aces_final.pdf (accessed February 17, 2015).

15 *An ACE Score of 6 and higher shortened:* D. W. Brown, R. F. Anda, et al., "Adverse Childhood Experiences and the Risk of Premature Mortality," *American Journal of Preventive Medicine* 37, no. 5 (November 2009), 389–96.

16 *Adults who faced early life stress show greater erosion:* I. Shalev, S. Entringer, P. D. Wadhwa, et al., "Stress and Telomere Biology: A Lifespan Perspective," *Psychoneuroendocrinoogy* 38, no. 9 (September 2013), 835–42. L. H. Price, H. T. Kao, D. E. Burgers, et al., "Telomeres and Early Life Stress: An Overview," *Biological Psychiatry* 73, no. 1 (January 2013), 15–23.

16 *For instance, children whose parents die:* M. Dong, W. H. Giles, V. J. Felitti, et al., "Insights into Causal Pathways for Ischemic Heart Disease: Adverse Childhood Experiences Study," *Circulation* 110, no. 13 (September 28, 2004), 1761–66; D. W. Brown, R. F. Anda, V. J. Felitti, et al., "Adverse Childhood Experiences Are Associated with the Risk of Lung Cancer: A Prospective Cohort Study," *BMC Public Health* 19, no. 10 (January 2010), 20; R. Anda, G. Tietjen, E. Schulman, et al., "Adverse Childhood Experiences and Frequent Headaches in Adults," *Headache* 50, no. 9 (October 2010), 1473–81; R. D. Goodwin, M. B. Stein, "Association Between Childhood Trauma and Physical Disorders Among Adults in the United States," *Psychological Medicine* 34, no. 3 (April 2004), 509–20; S. R. Dube, D. Fairweather, W. S. Pearson, et al., "Cumulative Childhood Stress and Autoimmune Diseases in Adults," *Psychosomatic Medicine* 71, no. 2 (February 2009), 243–50.

For more on the relationship between ACE Scores and specific diseases, see http://www.cdc.gov/ace/outcomes.htm (accessed February 19, 2013).

16 *They are more likely to develop cancer or have:* M. A. Bellis, K. Hughes, N. Leckenby, et al., "Measuring Mortality and the Burden of Adult Disease Associated with Adverse Childhood Experiences in England: A National Survey," *Journal of Public Health* (Oxford), August 30, 2014.

16 *Facing difficult circumstances in childhood increases:* C. Heim, U. M. Nater, E. Maloney, et al., "Childhood Trauma and Risk for Chronic Fatigue Syndrome: Association with Neuroendocrine Dysfunction," *Archives of General Psychiatry* 66, no. 1 (January 2009), 72–80. *Kids who lose a parent have triple the risk:* N. M. Melhem, M. Walker, G. Moritz et al., "Antecedents and Sequelae of Sudden Parental Death in Offspring and Surviving Caregivers," *Archives of Pediatrics and Adolescent Medicine* 162, no. 5 (May 2008), 403–10.

16 *Children whose parents divorce are twice as likely:* "Is There a Link Between Parental Divorce During Childhood and Stroke in Adulthood? Findings from a Population-Based Survey," presented by Esme Fuller-Thomson, PhD, and coauthored by Angela D. Dalton and Rukshan Mehta, on November 22, 2010, at the Gerontological Society of America (GSA) 63rd Annual Scientific Meeting. This paper is based on a representative community sample of more than 13,000 people from the 2005 Canadian Community Health Survey.

25 *The unifying principle of this:* To my knowledge, the concept that your biography becomes your biology was introduced into the field of holistic health by Caroline Myss and used in her teachings and books.

25 *For instance, in 2014, researchers at the University of Cambridge:* N. D. Walsh, T. Dalgleish, M. V. Lombardo, et al., "General and Specific Effects of Early Life Psychosocial Adversities on Adolescent Grey Matter Volume," *NeuroImage: Clinical* 4 (2014): 308–18, http://dx.doi.org/10.1016/j.nicl.2014.01.001.

26 *Brain imaging of these same kids:* Ibid.

26 *Because the CTQ lets respondents paint:* R. J. Herringa, R. M. Birn, P. L. Ruttle, et al., "Childhood Maltreatment Is Associated with Altered Fear Circuitry and Increased Internalizing Symptoms by Late Adolescence," *Proceedings of the National Academy of Sciences of the United States of America* 110, no. 47 (November 19, 2013), 19119–24.

27 *As Felitti observes, the years of "infancy":* V. J. Felitti and R. F. Anda, "The Relationship of Adverse Childhood Experiences to Adult Health, Well-Being, Social Function, and Health Care," in *The Effects of Early Life Trauma on Health and Disease: The Hidden Epidemic,* edited by R. Lanius, E. Vermetten, C. Pain, (New York: Cambridge University Press, 2010), Chapter 8.

Chapter Two: Different Adversities Lead to Similar Health Problems

31 *As Stanford professor Robert Sapolsky, PhD:* Robert Sapolsky, PhD, said this in the film *Killer Stress: A National Geographic Special,* and you can view a transcript here: http://tv.ark.com/transcript/killer_stress__a_national_geographic_special /1020/KTEH/Monday_April_12_2010/258324/ (accessed February 25, 2015).

31 *For example, adults under the stress of taking care of spouses:* J. K. Kiecolt-Glaser, K.

J. Preacher, R. C. MacCallum, et al., "Chronic Stress and Age-Related Increases in the Proinflammatory Cytokine IL-6," *Proceedings of the National Academy of Sciences of the United States of America,* 100, no. 15 (July 22, 2003), 9090–95.

31 *Likewise, if an adult sibling dies:* M. Rostila, J. Saarela, and I. Kawachi, "Mortality from Myocardial Infarction After the Death of a Sibling: A Nationwide Follow-up Study from Sweden," *Journal of the American Heart Association* 27, no. 2 (February 27, 2013), e000046.

31 *If you're pregnant and face a big, stressful event:* C. J. Hogue, C. B. Parker, M. Willinger, et al., "A Population-Based Case-Control Study of Stillbirth: The Relationship of Significant Life Events to the Racial Disparity for African Americans," *American Journal of Epidemiology* 177, no. 8 (April 15, 2013), 755-67; K. Wisborg, A. Barklin, M. Hedegaard, et al., "Psychological Stress During Pregnancy and Stillbirth: Prospective Study," *BJOG* 115, no. 7 (June 2008), 882–85.

31 *Encountering serious financial problems raises:* H. A. Fink, M. A. Kuskowski, and L. M. Marshall, "Association of Stressful Life Events with Incident Falls and Fractures in Older Men: The Osteoporotic Fractures in Men (MrOS) Study," *Age and Ageing* 43, no. 1 (January 2014), 103–8.

31 *A child's death triples a parent's chance:* J. Li C. Johansen, H. Brønnum-Hansen, et al., "The Risk of Multiple Sclerosis in Bereaved Parents: A Nationwide Cohort Study in Denmark," *Neurology* 62, no. 5 (March 9, 2004), 5, 726–29.

31 *States of intense emotional fear or loss can precipitate:* "Broken heart syndrome mimics heart attack symptoms. The condition usually strikes women during a time of extreme stress. However, the symptoms typically vanish without causing lasting harm," *Heart Advisor* 11, no. 4 (April 2008), 5, 7.

32 *ACE Scores are linked to a far greater likelihood of diseases including cancer:* C. Heim, U. M. Nater, E. Maloney, et al., "Childhood Trauma and Risk for Chronic Fatigue Syndrome: Association with Neuroendocrine Dysfunction," *Archives of General Psychiatry* 66, no. 1 (January 2009), 72–80; D. W. Brown, R. F. Anda, V. J. Felitti, et al., "Adverse Childhood Experiences Are Associated with the Risk of Lung Cancer: A Prospective Cohort Study," *BioMedCentral Public Health* 19, no. 10 (January 2010), 20; D. W. Brown, R. F. Anda, V. J. Felitti, et al., "Adverse Childhood Experiences and Frequent Headaches in Adults," *Headache* 50, no. 9 (October 2010), 1473-81; R. D. Goodwin and M. B. Stein, "Association Between Childhood Trauma and Physical Disorders Among Adults in the United States," *Psychological Medicine* 34, no. 3 (April 2004), 509–20; S. R. Dube, D. Fairweather, W. S. Pearson, et al., "Cumulative Childhood Stress and Autoimmune Diseases in Adults," *Psychosomatic Medicine* 71, no. 2 (February 2009), 243–50. For more on the relationship between ACE Scores and disease, see http://www.cdc.gov/ace/outcomes.htm (accessed February 20, 2015).

32 *The more categories of Adverse Childhood Experiences:* M. Dong, W. H. Giles , V. J. Felitti, et al., "Insights into Causal Pathways for Ischemic Heart Disease: Adverse Childhood Experiences Study," *Circulation* 110, no. 13 (September 28, 2004), 1761–66.

36 *In other words, when a child is young and his brain:* I've based this description of Michael Meaney's gene methylation theory on that provided in an article by Paul Tough, "The Poverty Clinic," *The New Yorker* (March 21, 2011), 25–30. For more

on how childhood adversity is associated with epigenetic alterations in the pro-moters of several genes in hippocampal neurons, see B. Labonté, M. Suderman, G. Maussion, et al., "Genome-Wide Epigenetic Regulation by Early Life Trauma," *Archives of General Psychiatry* 69, no. 7 (July 2012), 722–31.

36 *Kaufman found significant differences in epigenetic markers:* N. Weder. H. Zhang, K. Jensen, et al., "Child Abuse, Depression, and Methylation in Genes Involved with Stress, Neural Plasticity, and Brain Circuitry," *Journal of the American Academy of Child and Adolescent Psychiatry* 53, no. 4 (April 2014), 417–24.e5.

36 *Seth Pollak, PhD, professor of psychology and director:* S. E. Romens, J. McDonald, J. Svaren, et al., "Associations Between Early Life Stress and Gene Methylation in Children," *Child Development* (July 24, 2014). You can read more about Seth Pollak's recent work in the web article "Abuse Casts a Long Shadow by Changing Children's Genes," by Eleanor Nelsen, http://www.pbs.org/wgbh/nova/next/body/epigenetics-abuse (accessed February 15, 2015). Prior to Seth Pollak's work, Moshe Szyf and Michael Meaney at McGill University found in 2005 that rat pups raised by abusive mothers demonstrated epigenetic changes. M. J. Meaney and M. Szyf, "Environmental Programming of Stress Responses Through DNA Methylation: Life at the Interface Between a Dynamic Environment and a Fixed Genome," *Dialogues, Clinical Neuroscience* 7, no. 2 (2005), 103–23.

37 *"A crucial set of brakes are off":* According to Seth Pollak, PhD, it is important to note that in human epigenetic studies, "We can't really know for sure that what we have observed in children reflects this problem in the stress response system. Nonhuman animal studies measure the gene right from the brain (using the ani-mal brain tissue). We can't do that with children, of course, so we take the genes from blood. But blood is far away from the brain. If the gene we find in the blood is working the same as the gene in the brain, then we know our theory is true. However, if the gene functions differently in the blood than in the brain, we can't say the brake on the stress response system is broken. But we can say that the stress response system will affect the child's immune system. This means that stress-ex-posed children will be less able to fight off pathogens and will be more susceptible to illness. In fact, we have found this to be the case." For more on this, see E. A. Shirtcliff, C. L. Coe, and S. D. Pollak, "Early Childhood Stress Is Associated with Elevated Antibody Levels to Herpes Simplex Virus Type 1," *Proceedings of the National Academy of Sciences of the United States of America* 106, no. 8 (February 2009), 2963–67.

37 *This is only one of hundreds of genes that are damaged:* M. Suderman, P. O. McGowan, A. Sasaki, et al., "Conserved Epigenetic Sensitivity to Early Life Experience in the Rat and Human Hippocampus," *Proceedings of the National Academy of Sciences of the United States of America* 109, Suppl. 2 (October 16, 2012), 17266–72.

37 *Joan Kaufman and her colleagues discovered:* B. Z. Yang, H. Zhang, J. Kaufman, et al., "Child Abuse and Epigenetic Mechanisms of Disease Risk," *American Journal of Preventive Medicine* 44, no. 2 (February 2013), 101–17.

41 *According to ACE research, growing up with:* A. Gjelsvik, D. M. Dumont, A. Nunn, et al., "Adverse Childhood Events: Incarceration of Household Members and

Health-Related Quality of Life in Adulthood," *Journal of Health Care for the Poor and Underserved*, 25, no. 3 (August 2014), 1169–82.

41 *At the end of the three weeks, McCarthy's team:* C. G. Reich, M. E. Taylor, and M. M. McCarthy, "Differential Effects of Chronic Unpredictable Stress on Hippocampal CB1 Receptors in Male and Female Rats," *Behavioural Brain Research* 203, no. 2 (November 5, 2009), 264–69.

47 *According to the National Institute of Mental Health:* National Institute of Mental Health, Any Mental Illness (AMI) Among Adults, http://www.nimh.nih.gov/health/statistics/prevalence/any-mental-illness-ami-among-adults.shtml (accessed February 20, 2015).

47 *Twenty-three million adult Americans suffer from an alcohol:* "New Data Show Millions of Americans with Alcohol and Drug Addiction Could Benefit from Health Care," Partnership for Drug Free Kids (September 28, 2010), http://www.drugfree.org/untaxed/new-data-show-millions-of (accessed February 20, 2015).

48 *Thirty percent of those with an ACE Score of 3:* Robert Anda, MD, "The Health and Social Impact of Growing Up with Adverse Childhood Experiences," http://acestudy.org/files/Review_of_ACE_Study_with_references_summary_table_2_.pdf (accessed February 20, 2015).

48 *Sixteen percent of respondents to the Adverse Childhood Experience:* Vincent J. Felitti, MD, and Robert F. Anda, MD, "The Relationships of Adverse Childhood Experiences to Adult Health Status," (September 27, 2010), http://www.sanctuaryweb.com/PDFs/ACEs%20Handout%20&%20Pubs.pdf (accessed February 20, 2015).

48 *And 35 percent of men, versus nearly 60:* Ibid.

48 *The strongest precursor of adult depression:* D. P., C. L. Whitfield, V. J. Felitti, et al., "Adverse Childhood Experiences and the Risk of Depressive Disorders in Adulthood," *Journal of Affective Disorders* 82, no. 2 (October 2004), 217–25.

48 *Whether you are male or female, the loss of a parent:* N. M. Melhem, M. Walker, G. Moritz, et al., "Antecedents and Sequelae of Sudden Parental Death in Offspring and Surviving Caregivers," *Archives of Pediatrics and Adolescent Medicine* 162, no. 5 (May 2008), 403–10.

48 *Children who experienced severe trauma before the age of sixteen:* R. P. Bentall, S. Wickham, M. Shevlin, et al., "Do Specific Early-Life Adversities Lead to Specific Symptoms of Psychosis? A Study from the 2007 The Adult Psychiatric Morbidity Survey," *Schizophrenia Bulletin* 38, no. 4 (June 2012), 734–40.

48 *Most disturbing are the statistics on suicide:* Vincent J. Felitti, MD, and Robert F. Anda, MD, "The Relationships of Adverse Childhood Experiences to Adult Health Status," (September 27, 2010), http://www.sanctuaryweb.com/PDFs/ACEs%20Handout%20&%20Pubs.pdf (accessed February 20, 2015).

48 *Indeed, a person with an ACE Score of 4 or more is:* S. R. Dube, R. F. Anda, V. J. Felitti, et al., "Childhood Abuse, Household Dysfunction, and the Risk of Attempted Suicide Throughout the Life-Span: Findings from the Adverse Childhood Experiences Study," *Journal of the American Medical Association* 286, no. 24 (December 2001), 3089–96.

49 *That smaller brain volume may be due to a reduction:* M. A. Sheridan, N. A. Fox, C.

H. Zeanah, et al., "Variation in Neural Development as a Result of Exposure to Institutionalization Early in Childhood," *Proceedings of the National Academy of Sciences of the United States of America* 109, no. 32 (August 7, 2012), 12927–32.

51 *In a healthy brain, microglia control:* C. L. Cunningham, V. Martínez-Cerdeño, and S. C. Noctor, "Microglia Regulate the Number of Neural Precursor Cells in the Developing Cerebral Cortex," *Journal of Neuroscience* 33, no. 10 (March 6, 2013), 4216–33.

51 *They are essential in a healthy brain:* D. P. Schafer, E. K. Lehrman, A. G. Kautzman, et al., "Microglia Sculpt Postnatal Neural Circuits in an Activity and Complement-Dependent Manner," *Neuron* 74, no. 4 (May 24, 2012), 691–705.

51 *Indeed research suggests, says McCarthy:* A. Sierra, S. Beccari, I. Diaz-Aparicio, et al., "Surveillance, Phagocytosis, and Inflammation: How Never Resting Microglia Influence Adult Hippocampal Neurogenesis," *Neural Plasticity*, March 2014, 610343.

51 *The results have been stunning:* T. Kreisel, M. G. Frank, T. Licht, et al., "Dynamic Microglial Alterations Underlie Stress-Induced Depressive-like Behavior and Suppressed Neurogenesis," *Molecular Psychiatry* 19 (2014), 699–709.

52 *Dan Siegel, MD, child neuropsychiatrist:* Child psychiatrist Dan Siegel, MD, is the widely accepted scientific father of the field of interpersonal neurobiology. He is the author of a number of books, including *Brainstorm: The Power and Purpose of the Teenage Brain; Mindsight: The New Science of Personal Transformation;* and co-author, with Tina Payne Bryson, of *The Whole-Brain Child: 12 Revolutionary Strategies to Nurture Your Child's Developing Mind, Survive Everyday Parenting Struggles, and Help Your Family Thrive* and *No-Drama Discipline.*

53 *Imagine, hypothetically speaking:* This analogy is loosely drawn from a talk that Dan Siegel, MD, gave based on his book, *Brainstorm: The Power and Purpose of the Teenage Brain* at the Family Action Network in New York, New York, https://www.youtube.com/watch?v=kH-BO1rJXbQ (accessed February 20, 2015).

56 *It also sheds light on why, according to:* In 2012, an estimated 16 million adults aged eighteen or older in the United States had at least one major depressive episode in the past year, and an estimated 2.2 million adolescents aged twelve to seventeen in the United States had at least one major depressive episode in the past year. Added together, depression affects 18 million Americans, http://www.nimh.nih.gov/health/statistics/prevalence/major-depression-among-adults.shtml http://www.nimh.nih.gov/health/statistics/prevalence/major-depression-among-adolescents.shtml (accessed February 25, 2015).

56 *The World Health Organization recently cited depression:* World Health Organization, "Depression: A Hidden Burden," http://www.who.int/mental_health/management/depression/flyer_depression_2012.pdf (accessed February 20, 2015).

56 *The greater a patient's level of self-reported CFS symptoms:* Y. Nakatomi, K. Mizuno, A. Ishii, et al., "Neuroinflammation in Patients with Chronic Fatigue Syndrome/Myalgic Encephalomyelitis: An 11C-(R)-PK11195 PET Study," *Journal of Nuclear Medicine* 55, no. 6 (March 24, 2014), 945–50.

57 *This may also help to account for why it is that those:* C. Heim, U. M. Nater, E. Maloney, et al., "Childhood Trauma and Risk for Chronic Fatigue Syndrome: Association with Neuroendocrine Dysfunction," *Archives of General Psychiatry* 66, no. 1 (January 2009), 72–80.

Chapter Three: Why Do Some Suffer More than Others?

60 *Even those centenarians who have:* This understanding comes from the following online interview, as well as from an email exchange with Margery Silver on January 26, 2015: Norman Swan, "Interview with Margery Silver and Thomas Perls," September 14, 2008, http://centenariansecrets.blogspot.com/2008/09/interview-with-margery-silver-and.html (accessed February 20, 2015).

62 *But one time in ten, out of that despair:* Malcolm Gladwell, *David and Goliath: Underdogs, Misfits, and the Art of Battling Giants* (New York: Little, Brown, 2013); Robert Krulwich, "Successful Children Who Lost a Parent—Why Are There So Many of Them?," National Public Radio (October 16, 2013). www.npr.org/blogs/krulwich/2013/10/15/234737083/successful-children-who-lost-a-parent-why-are-there-so-many-of-them (accessed February 20, 2015).

62 *John F. Kennedy, whom biographers cite as:* You can read more on the PBS website, *American Experience, Biography: Rose Kennedy,* http://www.pbs.org/wgbh/amer icanexperience/features/biography/kennedys-bio-rose-fitzgerald/ Additional revelations about JFK's health appear in the following article: Robert Dallek, "The Medical Ordeals of JFK," *The Atlantic Monthly,* December 2002, http://www.the atlantic.com/magazine/archive/2002/12/the-medical-ordeals-of-jfk/305572/. Dallek was granted exclusive access to Kennedy's private papers for the years 1955 to 1963, including his X-rays and prescription drug records (accessed February 22, 2015).

63 *As Gladwell found, nine out of ten people:* Joe Nocera, "Malcolm Gladwell's 'David and Goliath,'" *The New York Times Sunday Book Review* (October 11, 2013), http://www.nytimes.com/2013/10/13/books/review/malcolm-gladwells-david-and-goliath.html?_r=0%20http:// (accessed February 20, 2015).

64 *In other words, those participants who had a score of 0:* M. D. Seery, R. J. Leo, E. A. Holman, et al., "Lifetime Exposure to Adversity Predicts Functional Impairment and Healthcare Utilization Among Individuals with Chronic Back Pain," *Pain* 150, no. 3 (September 2010), 507–15.

65 *And this same group was less likely to have a higher:* M. D. Seery, R. J. Leo, S. P. Lupien, et al., "An Upside to Adversity? Moderate Cumulative Lifetime Adversity Is Associated with Resilient Responses in the Face of Controlled Stressors," *Psychological Science* 24, no. 7 (July 1, 2013), 1181–89.

65 *This group also reported less emotional distress:* M. D. Seery, E. A. Holman, R. C. Silver, et al., "Whatever Does Not Kill Us: Cumulative Lifetime Adversity, Vulnerability, and Resilience," *Journal of Personality and Social Psychology* 99, no. 6 (December 2010), 1025–41.

66 *Recently Jack Shonkoff, MD, director of the Center on the Developing:* This discussion, hosted by The Forum at Harvard School of Public Health, was titled "The Toxic Stress of Early Childhood Adversity: Rethinking Health and Education Policy," February 7, 2012, http://developingchild.harvard.edu/resources/multimedia/lectures_and_presentations/hsph-forum/ (accessed February 20, 2015).

67 *This is the stress associated with chronic activation of systems:* Ibid.

68 *And 60 percent of these teens who said:* K. A. McLaughlin, J. Greif Green, M. J.

Gruber, et al., "Childhood Adversities and First Onset of Psychiatric Disorders in a National Sample of U.S. Adolescents" (2012), 1151–60.

72 *With someone to lean on, and with love:* Center on the Developing Child, Harvard University, "Key Concepts: Toxic Stress," http://developingchild.harvard.edu/index.php/key_concepts/toxic_stress_response/ (accessed February 20, 2015).

72 *Having supportive, responsive relationships with caring adults:* Ibid.

74 *Researchers at Emory University recently found that even when children:* B. Bradley, T. A. Davis, A. P. Wingo, et al., "Family Environment and Adult Resilience: Contributions of Positive Parenting and the Oxytocin Receptor Gene," *European Journal of Psychotraumatology* (September 18, 2013), 4.

75 *This Sensitivity Gene exists in three variants:* Gene variants are also known as gene alleles. The term *allele*—which comes from the word *allelomorph,* meaning "other form"—refers to the different forms any one gene can take. For instance, our gene alleles usually code for our red blood cells to have a round, concave shape. But if there is a mutation in that gene, which causes another allele to be expressed, a red blood cell might be shaped, instead, in the form of a sickle—causing sickle-cell anemia.

76 *People with this Sensitivity Gene variant who experience:* K. Karg, M. Burmeister, S. Sen, et al., "The Serotonin Transporter Promoter Variant (5-HTTLPR), Stress, and Depression Meta-Analysis Revisited: Evidence of Genetic Moderation," *Archives of General Psychiatry* 68, no. 5 (May 2011), 444–54. In the study, Srijan Sen, MD, PhD, assistant professor of psychiatry at the University of Michigan Medical School, and his colleagues examined fifty-four studies done between 2001 and 2010 looking at 41,000 individuals—the largest analysis ever done of the relationship between individuals' serotonin genetic makeup and how well they were able to bounce back from adversity.

76 *The reason is this: the Sensitivity Gene influences:* M. Aquilera, B. Arias, M. Wichers et al., "Early Adversity and 5-HTT/BDNF Genes: New Evidence of Gene-Environment Interactions on Depressive Symptoms in a General Population," *Psychological Medicine* 39, no. 9 (September 2009), 1425–32.

77 *These same kids also showed signs of cognitive:* M. Owens, I. M. Goodyer, P. Wilkinson, et al., "5-HTTLPR and Early Childhood Adversities Moderate Cognitive and Emotional Processing in Adolescence," *PLoS One* 7, no. 11 (2012), e48482.

77 *Seventy-five percent of kids with the stress-reactive variant:* D. Albert, D. W. Belsky, M. Crowley, et al., "Can Genetics Predict Response to Complex Behavioral Interventions? Evidence from a Genetic Analysis of the Fast Track Randomized Control Trial," *Journal of Policy Analysis and Management* (January 2, 2015), doi: 10.1002/pam.21811.

80 *Even later efforts in adulthood to reshape:* J. Belsky and M. Pluess, "Beyond Diathesis Stress: Differential Susceptibility to Environmental Influences," *Psychological Bulletin* 135, no. 6 (2009), 885–908; J. Belsky, "Variation in Susceptibility to Rearing Influences: An Evolutionary Argument," *Psychological Inquiry* 8 (1997), 182–86; J. Belsky, "Theory Testing, Effect-Size Evaluation, and Differential Susceptibility to Rearing Influence: The Case of Mothering and Attachment," *Child Development* 68, no. 4 (1997), 598–600; J. Belsky, "Differential Susceptibility to Rearing Influ-

ences: An Evolutionary Hypothesis and Some Evidence," in *Origins of the Social Mind: Evolutionary Psychology and Child Development*, edited by B. Ellis and D. Bjorklund (New York: Guildford, 2005), 139–63.

80 *When "sensitive" children experience a supportive:* S. E. Taylor, B. M. Way, W. T. Welch, et al., "Early Family Environment, Current Adversity, the Serotonin Transporter Promoter Polymorphism, and Depressive Symptomatology," *Biologial Psychiatry* 60, no. 7 (October 1, 2006), 671–76.

80 *They become even more likely than other people to develop positive:* David Dobbs, "The Science of Success," *The Atlantic*, December 2009, accessed February 20, 2015). In this article Dobbs describes how Stephen Suomi, PhD, a rhesus-monkey researcher who heads a set of laboratories at the National Institutes of Health's Laboratory of Comparative Ethology, was the first researcher to work with the three different forms of the serotonin gene, and to conduct "gene-by-environment" studies to determine their effect. Suomi found that monkeys who carried the supposedly risky short/short gene variant, and who also had nurturing mothers, were better at making friends when they were young, made strong alliances as they grew older and knew how to utilize them, and handled larger group conflicts well. They rose higher in their respective hierarchies. Despite their short serotonin gene variant, they were the most successful monkeys in the troop. The implication, then, is that some brains are more plastic than others, and are therefore more affected by both positive and negative effects of supportive or unsupportive environments.

81 *Not surprisingly, those who had experienced a lot:* A. Keller, K. Litzelman, L. E. Wisk, et al., "Does the Perception that Stress Affects Health Matter? The Association with Health and Mortality," *Health Psychology* 31, no. 5 (2012), 677–84.

81 *In fact, she points out, this latter group:* Kelly McGonigal's TED Talk on the upside of stress can be found here: Kelly McGonigal, PhD, "How to Make Stress Your Friend," TEDGlobal 2013 (June 2013), http://www.ted.com/talks/kelly_mcgonigal_how_to_make_stress_your_friend (accessed April 7, 2014).

84 *When something traumatic occurs, the hormone noradrenaline:* E. S. Faber, A. J. Delaney, J. M. Power et al., "Modulation of SK Channel Trafficking by Beta Adrenoceptors Enhances Excitatory Synaptic Transmission and Plasticity in the Amygdala," *Journal of Neuroscience* 28, no. 43 (October 22, 2008), 10803–13.

84 *Each time we remember an incident of childhood adversity:* J. Debiec, L. Díaz-Mataix, D. E. Bush, et al., "The Amygdala Encodes Specific Sensory Features of an Aversive Reinforcer," *Nature Neuroscience* 13, no. 5 (May 2010), 536–37.

85 *When we mentally revisit an event, we are always:* This understanding is based on a series of interviews with Ruth Lanius, MD, PhD, on November 1, 2013, and November 11, 2013.

85 *But to some degree, memory plays hoaxes on us all:* H. Schmolck, E. A. Buffalo, and L. R. Squire, "Memory Distortions Develop over Time: Recollections of the O. J. Simpson Trial Verdict After 15 and 32 Months," *Psychological Science* 11, no. 1 (January 2000), 39–45.

85 *Our brains construct a world that no one else can see:* Michael S. Roth, author of *Memory, Trauma, and History: Essays on Living with the Past*, and president of

Wesleyan University, wrote this in his essay about Oliver Sacks's book *Hallucinations* in a review titled "A Neurologist in the Sky with Diamonds," *Washington Post*, December 30, 2012; (accessed February 21, 2015).

87 *As the Buddhist teacher Thich Nhat Hanh says:* Priscilla quotes Thich Nhat Hanh in her book *Learning to Breathe: My Yearlong Quest to Bring Calm to My Life* (New York: Free Press, 2011), 79.

87 *It takes two hundred milliseconds for the amygdala to compute:* Linda Graham, MFT, talks about this in a Clinical Conversation at the Community Institute for Psychotherapy, in a talk titled "The Neuroscience of Attachment," first presented Fall 2008. You can find a transcript of her talk at http://lindagraham-mft.net/re sources/published-articles/the-neuroscience-of-attachment/ (accessed February 21, 2015).

Chapter Four: The Female Brain on Adversity: The Link to Autoimmune Disease, Depression, and Anxiety

96 *When Vincent Felitti first published his Adverse Childhood Experience:* V. J. Felitti and R. F. Anda, "The Relationship of Adverse Childhood Experiences to Adult Medical Disease, Psychiatric Disorders, and Sexual Behavior: Implications for Healthcare," in *The Effects of Early Life Trauma on Health and Disease: The Hidden Epidemic,* edited by R. Lanius, E. Vermetten, and C. Pain (New York: Cambridge University Press, 2010), Chapter 8, p. 77.

97 *Fairweather looked at each ACE study:* S. R. Dube, D. Fairweather, W. S. Pearson, et al., "Cumulative Childhood Stress and Autoimmune Diseases in Adults," *Psychosomatic Medicine* 71, no. 2 (February 2009), 243–50.

98 *For instance, a woman with three Adverse Childhood Experiences:* Ibid.

99 *Indeed, if you are diagnosed with one autoimmune disease:* G. S. Cooper, M. L. Bynum, E. C. Somers, "Recent Insights in the Epidemiology of Autoimmune Diseases: Improved Prevalence Estimates and Understanding of Clustering of Diseases," *Journal of Autoimmunity* 33, nos. 3–4 (November–December 2009), 197–207.

99 *And, says Fairweather, "80 percent of these patients":* D. L. Jacobson, S. J. Gange, N. R. Rose, et al. "Epidemiology and Estimated Population Burden of Selected Autoimmune Diseases in the United States," *Clinical Immunology Immunopathology* 84, no. 3 (September 1997), 223–43.

100 *Autoimmune disease is one of the top ten leading:* American Autoimmune Related Diseases Association, Inc., press release for National Autoimmune Disease Awareness Month, March 22, 2014, http://myemail.constantcontact.com/Spread-the-news-about-autoimmune-disease.html?soid=1115217054950&aid=HHLCBw3ETFs (accessed April 9, 2014).

100 *Although Fairweather, Felitti, and Anda did not include multiple sclerosis:* C. Spitzer, M. Bouchain, L. Y. Winkler, et al., "Childhood Trauma in Multiple Sclerosis: A Case-Control Study," *Psychosomatic Medicine* 74, no. 3 (April 2012), 312–18.

103 *Recent studies show that the average woman sees five doctors:* American Autoimmune Related Diseases Association, Inc., press release for National Autoimmune Disease Awareness Month, March 22, 2014, http://myemail.constantcontact.com/Spread-

the-news-about-autoimmune-disease.html?soid=1115217054950&aid=HHLC-Bw3ETFs (accessed April 9, 2014).

103 *Girls not only face more adverse experiences:* J. L. Hamilton, J. P. Stange, L. Y. Abramson, et al., "Stress and the Development of Cognitive Vulnerabilities to Depression Explain Sex Differences in Depressive Symptoms During Adolescence," *Clinical Psychological Science* (October 2, 2014).

104 *This, in turn, puts them more at risk:* Bessel van der Kolk, MD, *The Body Keeps the Score: Brain, Mind, and Body in the Healing of Trauma* (New York: Viking, 2014), 126–27.

107 *Moreover, maltreatment's effect on girls' frontal lobe:* R. J. Herringa, R. M. Birn, P. L. Ruttle, et al., "Childhood Maltreatment Is Associated with Altered Fear Circuitry and Increased Internalizing Symptoms by Late Adolescence," *Proceedings of the National Academy of Sciences of the United States of America* 110, no. 47 (November 2013), 19119–24.

108 *Boys, on the other hand, were more likely to show decreases:* E. F. Edmiston, F. Wang, C. M. Mazure, et al., "Corticostriatal-limbic Gray Matter Morphology in Adolescents with Self-Reported Exposure to Childhood Maltreatment," *Archives of Pediatrics and Adolescent Medicine* 165, no. 12 (December 2011), 1069–77.

110 *Neuroinflammation disrupted specific neural circuits:* J. Czerniawski and J. F. Guzowski, "Acute Neuroinflammation Impairs Context Discrimination Memory and Disrupts Pattern Separation Processes in Hippocampus," *Journal of Neuroscience* 34, no. 37 (September 10, 2014), 12470–80.

111 *Boys with this gene variant who experience childhood trauma:* C. Heim, B. Bradley, T. C. Mletzko, et al., "Effect of Childhood Trauma on Adult Depression and Neuroendocrine Function: Sex-Specific Moderation by CRH Receptor 1 Gene," *Frontiers in Behavioral Neuroscience* 3 (November 2009), 6;3:41.

112 *Researchers at the Medical University of South Carolina:* S. M. DeSantis, N. L. Baker, S. E. Back, et al., "Gender Differences in the Effect of Early Life Trauma on Hypothalamic-Pituitary-Adrenal Axis Functioning," *Depression and Anxiety* 28, no. 5 (May 2011), 383–92.

113 *Typically, they are the most difficult patients:* V. J. Felitti and R. F. Anda, "The Relationship of Adverse Childhood Experiences to Adult Medical Disease, Psychiatric Disorders, and Sexual Behavior: Implications for Healthcare," in *The Effects of Early Life Trauma on Health and Disease: the Hidden Epidemic,* edited by R. Lanius, E. Vermetten, and C. Pain (New York: Cambridge University Press, 2010), Chapter 8, 78.

Chapter Five: The Good Enough Family

114 *Ninety-one percent of men who, decades earlier:* L. G. Russel and G. E. Schwartz, "Feelings of Parental Caring Predict Health Status in Midlife: A 35-Year Follow-up of the Harvard Mastery of Stress Study," *Journal of Behavioral Medicine* 20, no. 1 (February 1997), 1–13.

115 *This was true regardless of family medical history:* L. G. Russel and G. E. Schwartz, "Narrative Descriptions of Parental Love and Caring Predict Health Status in

Midlife: A 35-Year Follow-up of the Harvard Mastery of Stress Study," *Alternative Therapies in Health and Medicine* 2, no. 6 (November 1996), 55–62.

123 *The work of Robin Karr-Morse:* Robin Karr-Morse is coauthor with Meredith S. Wiley of the books *Scared Sick: The Role of Childhood Trauma in Adult Disease* (New York: Basic Books, 2012) and *Ghosts in the Nursery: Tracing the Roots of Violence* (New York: Grove Press, 2013).

123 *When this kind of emotional trauma happens routinely:* This understanding comes from my email conversations with Robin Karr-Morse as well as from this interview: Thomas Rogers, "How Stress is Really Hurting Our Kids, *Salon* (January 2, 2012), http://www.salon.com/2012/01/02/how_stress_is_really_hurting_our_kids/ (accessed May 15, 2014).

124 *If Mom has a flu during certain windows of pregnancy:* R. E. Kneeland and S. H. Fatemi, "Viral Infection, Inflammation and Schizophrenia," *Progress in Neuropsychopharmacology and Biological Psychiatry* 42 (April 5, 2013), 35–48.

124 *These effects last for generations:* P. Dominguez-Salas, S. E. Moore, M. S. Baker, et al., "Maternal Nutrition at Conception Modulates DNA Methylation of Human Metastable Epialleles," *Nature Communications* 5 (April 29, 2014), 3746; Assad Meymandi, MD, PhD, "The Science of Epigenetics," *Psychiatry* (Edgmont) 7, no. 3 (March 2010), 40–41.

125 *Even more startling, this anxious behavior:* Inna Gaisler-Salomon, "Inheriting Stress," *The New York Times Sunday Review* (March 7, 2014), http://www.nytimes.com/2014/03/09/opinion/sunday/can-children-inherit-stress.html (accessed February 22, 2015).

125 *Studies show that merely observing another person:* V. Engert, F. Plessow, R. Miller, et al., "Cortisol Increase in Empathic Stress Is Modulated by Social Closeness and Observation Modality," *Psychoneuroendocrinology*, April 17, 2014.

126 *These infants' heart rates went up:* S. F. Waters, T. V. West, and W. B. Mendes, "Stress Contagion: Physiological Covariation Between Mothers and Infants," *Psychological Science* 25, no. 4 (April 2014), 934–42.

127 *Babies whose parents argued a lot at home:* A. M. Graham, P. A. Fisher, and J. H. Pfeifer, "What Sleeping Babies Hear: A Functional MRI Study of Interparental Conflict and Infants' Emotion Processing," *Psychological Science* 24, no. 5 (May 2013), 782–99.

127 *For instance, kids whose moms suffer from anxiety:* C. U. Rask, E. Ørnbøl, E. M. Olsen, et al., "Infant Behaviors Are Predictive of Functional Somatic Symptoms at Ages Five to Seven Years: Results from the Copenhagen Child Cohort CCC2000," *Journal of Pediatrics* 162, no. 2 (February 2013), 335–42.

128 *Nor did they learn from Grace:* T. Dix, A. Moed, and E. R. Anderson, "Mothers' Depressive Symptoms Predict Both Increased and Reduced Negative Reactivity: Aversion Sensitivity and the Regulation of Emotion," *Psychological Science* 25, no. 7 (May 2014), 1353–61.

128 *These teens who didn't learn to calm themselves:* S. E. Anderson, R. A. Gooze, S. Lemeshow, et al., "Quality of Early Maternal-Child Relationship and Risk of Adolescent Obesity," *Pediatrics* 129, no. 1 (January 2012), 132–40.

129 *In fact, a nurturing mother offsets:* G. E. Miller, M. E. Lachman, E. Chen, et al.,

"Pathways to Resilience: Maternal Nurturance as a Buffer Against the Effects of Childhood Poverty on Metabolic Syndrome at Midlife," *Psychological Science* 22, no. 12 (December 2011), 1591–99.

130 *The victims of bullying had higher CRP levels:* W. E. Copeland, D. Wolke, S. T. Lereya, et al., "Childhood Bullying Involvement Predicts Low-Grade Systemic Inflammation into Adulthood," *Proceedings of the National Academy of Sciences in the United States of America* 111, no. 21 (May 27, 2014), 7570–75.

130 *Other studies show that children who experience bullying:* W. E. Copeland, D. Wolke, A. Angold, et al., "Adult Psychiatric Outcomes of Bullying and Being Bullied by Peers in Childhood and Adolescence," *JAMA Psychiatry* 70, no. 4 (April 2013), 419–26.

130 *Social pain, the kind that occurs if, say:* G. Novembre, M. Zanon, and G. Silani, "Empathy for Social Exclusion Involves the Sensory-Discriminative Component of Pain: A Within-Subject fMRI Study," *Social Cognitive & Affective Neuroscience* 10, no. 2 (February 2015), 153–64.

130 *In one study, which followed eight hundred kids:* P. E. Gustafsson, U. Janlert, T. Theorell et al., "Do Peer Relations in Adolescence Influence Health in Adulthood? Peer Problems in the School Setting and the Metabolic Syndrome in Middle-Age," *PLoS One* 7, no. 6 (2012), e39385.

130 *A recent SAFE survey found that:* Stomp Out Bullying, "About Bullying and Cyber Bullying," http://www.stompoutbullying.org/index.php/information-and-resources/about-bullying-and-cyberbullying (accessed January 14, 2015).

131 *Almost half of all kids reported fearing:* Bullying Statistics, "School Bullying Statistics," http://www.bullyingstatistics.org/content/school-bullying-statistics.html (accessed January 14, 2015).

131 *Disturbingly, about 80 percent of all high school:* Ibid.

131 *And over three-quarters of children who had emotional:* C. D. Bethell, P. Newacheck, E. Hawes, et al. Adverse Childhood Experiences: Assessing the Impact on Health and School Engagement and the Mitigating Role of Resilience. *Health Affairs*, 33, no. 12 (2014):2106-2115.

131 *Other studies have shown that children with a single ACE Score are ten times:* N. J. Burke, J. L. Hellman, B. G. Scott, et al., "The Impact of Adverse Childhood Experiences on an Urban Pediatric Population," 35, no. 6 (June 2011), 408–13.

131 *Teachers may suggest that these children be treated for ADHD:* Laura K. Kerr, PhD, "ADHD Symptoms? Psychologists, Psychiatrists Should Consider Child Maltreatment as the Cause Before Prescribing Meds" (March 6, 2013), ACEsTooHigh .Org, http://acestoohigh.com/2013/03/06/adhd-symptoms-psychologists-psy chiatrists-should-consider-child-maltreatment-as-the-cause-before-prescribing-meds/ (accessed January 14, 2015).

132 *Recently, the American Psychological Association:* American Psychological Association, "American Psychological Association Survey Shows Teen Stress Rivals That of Adults" (February 11, 2014), http://www.apa.org/news/press/releases/2014/02/teen-stress.aspx (accessed May 19, 2014).

133 *It's not surprising that, in the past decade, rates of "test anxiety":* N. Von der Embse, J. Barterian, and N. Segool, "Test Anxiety Interventions for Children and

Adolescents: A Systematic Review of Treatment Studies from 2000–2010," *Psychology in the Schools*, Vol. 50, Issue 1(Hoboken, NJ: Wiley Periodicals, Inc., 2013), 57-71. Authors write, "High-stakes tests have played an increasingly important role in how student achievement and school effectiveness are measured. Test anxiety has risen with the use of tests in educational decision making." S. King, C. T. Chambers, A. Huguet, et al., "The Epidemiology of Chronic Pain in Children and Adolescents Revisited: A Systematic Review," *Pain* 152, no. 12 (December 2011), 2729–38.

137 *Ruth Lanius, MD, PhD, is a neuroscientist and professor:* Ruth Lanius is also a coeditor of *The Impact of Early Life Trauma on Health and Disease: The Hidden Epidemic* (New York: Cambridge University Press, 2010).

139 *People who lost a parent early in life experienced:* S. C. Bunce et al., "When Positive Becomes Negative—ERP Evidence for Differential Processing of Affective Stimuli in Subjects with Parental Loss," *Psychophysiology*, 33 (1996), 26–26. Press release: "Unconscious Fear of Intimacy Linked to Early Parental Loss," *Michigan News* (May 21, 1997), http://ns.umich.edu/new/releases/1542-unconscious-fear-of-intimacy-linked-to-early-parental-loss (accessed 10, 2014).

139 *Other research shows that kids who lost a parent:* J. Ellis, C. Dowrick, and M. Lloyd-Williams, "The Long-Term Impact of Early Parental Death: Lessons from a Narrative Study," *Journal of the Royal Society of Medicine* 106, no. 2 (February 2013), 57–67.

142 *And this experience—being seen and known:* Linda Graham, MFT, talked about this in Clinical Conversation at the Community Institute for Psychotherapy in a talk titled "The Neuroscience of Attachment," first presented Fall 2008. You can find a transcript of her talk here at, http://lindagraham-mft.net/resources/published-articles/the-neuroscience-of-attachment/ (accessed February 21, 2015).

143 *Not surprisingly, these kids who'd had secure attachments:* In this study, researchers evaluated parents' interactions with children when they were very young. For the next twenty years, they followed those children who had demonstrated secure attachment to their moms, as well as those who'd shown less attachment. When the study participants became young adults, they were asked to bring their romantic partners to the lab and discuss a topic they often disagreed about heatedly. Couples argued with each other for ten minutes. For the four minutes following the argument, researchers evaluated how able participants were to recover from their negative feelings and to put the disagreement behind them. J. E. Salvatore, S. I. Kuo, R. D. Steele, et al., "Recovering from Conflict in Romantic Relationships: A Developmental Perspective," *Psychological Science* 22, no. 3 (March 2011), 376–83.

143 *Parents who were warm, consistent, not overreactive:* D. C. Kerr, D. M. Capaldi, K. C. Pears, et al., "A Prospective Three Generational Study of Fathers' Constructive Parenting: Influences from Family of Origin, Adolescent Adjustment, and Offspring Temperament," *Developmental Psychology* 45, no. 5 (September 2009), 1257–75.

144 *But men who had enjoyed a good relationship:* M. H. Mallers, S. T. Charles, S. D.

Neupert, et al., "Perceptions of Childhood Relationships with Mother and Father: Daily Emotional and Stressor Experiences in Adulthood," *Developmental Psychology*, 46, no. 6 (November 2010), 1651–61.

144 *In a twenty-five-year study, researchers followed boys:* D. C. Kerr, D. M. Capaldi, K. C. Pears, et al., "A Prospective Three Generational Study of Fathers' Constructive Parenting: Influences from Family of Origin, Adolescent Adjustment, and Offspring Temperament," *Developmental Psychology* 45, no. 5 (September 2009), 1257–75.

145 *As attachment researcher Louis Cozolino:* Louis J. Cozolino, *The Neuroscience of Human Relationships: Attachment and the Developing Social Brain* (New York: Norton, 2006), 7.

Chapter Six: Beginning Your Healing Journey

152 *You may not remember them but you still relive them:* This understanding is based on a series of interviews with Ruth Lanius, MD, PhD, on November 1, 2013, and November 11, 2013.

154 *The resilience survey below is based on resilience research:* This questionnaire was developed by the early childhood service providers, pediatricians, psychologists, and health advocates of Southern Kennebec Healthy Start, Augusta, Maine, in 2006, and updated in February 2013. Two psychologists in the group, Mark Rains and Kate McClinn, came up with the fourteen statements with editing suggestions by the other members of the group. The scoring system was modeled after the ACE Study questions. The content of the questions was based on a number of research studies from the literature over the past forty years including that of Emmy Werner and others. Its purpose is limited to parenting education. It was not developed for research. ACEsTooHigh News, "Got Your ACE Score? (and, at the end, What's Your Resilience Score?)," http://acestoohigh.com/got-your-ace-score/.

157 *According to Jane Stevens, journalist and founder:* Jane Stevens is finishing a book about how people, organizations, agencies, and communities are using ACEs research to solve our most intractable problems—e.g., eliminate school suspensions and expulsions, stop domestic violence, get the homeless back on their feet—and allow us to spend money in different ways.

158 *Studies show that writing about stressful experiences:* J. M. Smyth, A. A. Stone, A. Hurewitz, et al., "Effects of Writing About Stressful Experiences on Symptom Reduction in Patients with Asthma or Rheumatoid Arthritis: A Randomized Trial," *JAMA* 281, no. 14 (April 1999), 1304–9.

158 *Write continuously for twenty minutes a day:* James W. Pennebaker, PhD, is Regents Centennial Professor and Chair of the Department of Psychology at the University of Texas at Austin and author of several books, including *Writing to Heal: A Guided Journal for Recovering from Trauma and Emotional Upheaval* (Oakland, CA: New Harbinger Publications 2004). You can read more about his instructions on how to write to heal in this article: James Pennebaker, PhD., "Writing to Heal," The University of Texas at Austin at http://www.utexas.edu/features/archive/2005/writing.html (accessed August 12, 2014).

158 *For instance, when students were asked to write to heal:* J. M. Smyth, J. R. Hockemeyer,

K. E. Heron, et al., "Prevalence, Type, Disclosure, and Severity of Adverse Life Events in College Students," *Journal of the American College of Health* 57, no. 1 (July–August 2008), 69–76; J. W. Pennebaker, S. D. Gosling, and J. D. Ferrell, "Daily Online Testing in Large Classes: Boosting College Performance While Reducing Achievement Gaps," *PLoS One* 8, no. 11 (November 2013), e79774.

158 *When individuals wrote about emotional upheavals:* J. W. Pennebaker, J. K. Kiecolt-Glaser, and R. Glaser, "Disclosure of Traumas and Immune Function: Health Implications for Psychotherapy," *Journal of Consulting and Clinical Psychology* 56, no. 2 (April 1988), 239–45.

158 *Researchers at Carnegie Mellon found that the simple act:* K. S. Kassam and W. B. Mendes, "The Effects of Measuring Emotion: Physiological Reactions to Emotional Situations Depend on Whether Someone Is Asking," *PLoS One* 8, no. 7 (June 5, 2013), e64959. Karim Kassam, PhD, assistant professor of social and decision sciences at Carnegie Mellon, says that what was most impressive was the fact that "a subtle manipulation had a big impact on people's physiological response. Essentially, we're asking people how they're feeling and finding that doing so has a sizable impact on their cardiovascular response."

160 *"And so I asked her, what happened when you were:* Quotes from Bernie Siegel, MD, which appear in this book are drawn from my phone conversations with him and through email exchanges.

161 *Individuals who practiced mindfulness meditation:* P. Kaliman, M. J. Alvarez-López, M. Cosín-Tomás, "Rapid Changes in Histone Deacetylases and Inflammatory Gene Expression in Expert Meditators," *Psychoneuroendocrinology* 40 (February 2014), 96–107; Researcher Richard Davidson, PhD, professor of psychology and psychiatry at the University of Wisconsin-Madison and author of *The Emotional Life of Your Brain: How Its Unique Patterns Affect the Way You Think, Feel, and Live— and How You Can Change Them* (New York: Penguin, 2012), calls mindfulness a "neurally inspired behavioral intervention" that serves to help change the brain.

161 *Dr. Ryan Herringa, assistant professor:* Ryan Herringa, MD, PhD, is the assistant professor of Child and Adolescent Psychiatry at the University of Wisconsin and director of the Herringa Lab.

162 *When you become aware of your breath:* C. E. Kerr, M. D. Sacchet, S. W. Lazar, et al., "Mindfulness Starts with the Body: Somatosensory Attention and Top-Down Modulation of Cortical Alpha Rhythms in Mindfulness Meditation," *Frontiers in Human Neuroscience* 7 (February 13, 2013), 12.

162 T. Magyari, "Teaching mindfulness to women with complex trauma" in *Mindfulness-Oriented Interventions for Trauma: Integrating Contemplative Practices*, edited by V. M. Follette, J. Briere, D. Rozelle, J. W. Hopper, D. I. Rome (New York: Guildford Press, 2015), 143.

162 *In another study, people who took an eight-week mindfulness-based stress reduction:* B. K. Hölzel, J. Carmody, M. Vangel, et al., "Mindfulness Practice Leads to Increases in Regional Brain Gray Matter Density," *Psychiatry Research* 191, no. 1 (January 30, 2011), 36–43.

162 *MBSR training (which includes twenty-six hours:* O. Singleton, B. K. Hölzel, and M. Vangel, "Change in Brainstem Gray Matter Concentration Following a Mindfulness-

Notes

Based Intervention Is Correlated with Improvement in Psychological Well-Being," *Frontiers in Human Neuroscience* 8 (February 18, 2014), 33.

163 *To establish a daily meditation practice:* Tara Brach is also the author of *True Refuge: Finding Peace and Freedom in Your Own Awakened Heart* (New York: Bantam, 2013) and *Radical Acceptance: Embracing Your Life with the Heart of a Buddha* (New York: Bantam, 2003).

164 *Notice the difference between any thought:* You can find out more about Tara Brach, PhD, and get instructions on how to meditate at http://www.tarabrach.com/howtomeditate.html (accessed January 17, 2015).

171 *And the third is integration, the ability:* This understanding emerges from an interview with Daniel J. Siegel, MD, on October 16, 2015, as well as email exchanges and material from his book *Brainstorm: The Power and Purpose of the Teenage Brain* (New York: Penguin, 2014), 40, 111.

171 *"Mindsight enables us to go beyond":* Ibid, 41, 42.

171 *You can simply start where you are by regularly:* Ibid, 42, 43.

172 *What feelings are inside you?:* Ibid, 47

172 *"Ions flowing in and out of the membranes":* Ibid, 46

172 *Charles Raison, MD, mind-body medicine researcher:* T. W. Pace, L. T. Negi, B. Dodson-Lavelle, et al., "Engagement with Cognitively Based Compassion Training Is Associated with Reduced Salivary C-Reactive Protein from Before to After Training in Foster Care Program Adolescents," *Psychoneuroendocrinology* 38, no. 2 (February 2013), 294–99.

172 *In high-security prisons where inmates learned:* NPR, "At End-of-the Line Prison, an Unlikely Escape" (February 8, 2011), http://www.npr.org/2011/02/08/133505880/at-end-of-the-line-prison-an-unlikely-escape (accessed February 23, 2015).

174 *Forgiveness, Kornfield says:* Quotes are taken from a talk called "The Ancient Heart of Forgiveness" that Jack Kornfield gave on how we can tap into the human capacity for forgiveness, https://www.youtube.com/watch?v=yiRP-Q4mMtk (accessed August 28, 2014).

175 *One of my favorite forgiveness practices is a four-step:* This is a condensed excerpt of "Forgiveness Meditation" and it appears here with his permission. You can see a longer version in Dr. Gordon's book *Unstuck: Your Guide to the Seven-Stage Journey Out of Depression* (New York: Penguin, 2008), 296–98.

177 *These areas of the brain go offline during:* D. L. Cohen, N. Wintering, V. Tolles, et al., "Cerebral Blood Flow Effects of Yoga Training: Preliminary Evaluation of Four Cases, *Journal of Alternative and Complementary Medicine* 15, no. 1 (January 2009), 9–14.

178 *When you don't have enough GABA:* C. C. Streeter, J. E. Jensen, R. M. Perlmutter, et al., "Yoga Asana Sessions Increase Brain GABA Levels: A Pilot Study," *Journal of Alternative and Complementary Medicine* 13, no. 4 (May 2007), 419–26.

181 *This gut "microbiome" determines the state,* http://www.apa.org/monitor/2012/09/gut-feeling.aspx (accessed August 28, 2014).

182 *Some organisms in the gut might prove useful:* J. A. Bravo, P. Forsythe, M. V. Chew, et al., "Ingestion of Lactobacillus Strain Regulates Emotional Behavior and Central

GABA Receptor Expression in a Mouse via the Vagus Nerve," *Proceedings of the National Academy of Sciences United States of America* 108, no. 38 (September 20, 2011), 16050–55.

182 *According to gastroenterologist Emeran Mayer, MD:* (accessed February 23, 2015). See more in these two studies: M. Fleshner , "The Gut Microbiota: A New Player in the Innate Immune Stress Response?," *Brain, Behavior, and Immunity* 25, no. 3 (March 2011), 395–96; and M. T. Bailey, S. E. Dowd, J. D. Galley, et al., "Exposure to a Social Stressor Alters the Structure of the Intestinal Microbiota: Implications for Stressor-Induced Immunomodulation," *Brain, Behavior, and Immunity* 25, no. 3 (March 2011), 397–407.

184 *For instance, having strong social ties helps to improve:* M. Epplein, Y. Zheng, W. Zheng, et al., "Quality of Life After Breast Cancer Diagnosis and Survival," *Journal of Clinical Oncology* 29, no. 4 (February 1, 2011), 406–12; R. F. Brown, C. C. Tennant, M. Sharrock, et. al., "Relationship Between Stress and Relapse in Multiple Sclerosis: Part II. Direct and Indirect Relationships," *Multiple Sclerosis Journal* 12, no. 4 (August 2006), 465–75.

184 *In part, that's because positive, supportive interactions:* J. P. Gouin, C. S. Carter, H. Pournajafi-Nazarloo, et al., "Marital Behavior, Oxytocin, Vasopressin, and Wound Healing," *Psychoneuroendocrinology* 35, no. 7 (August 2010), 1082–90.

Chapter Seven: Seeking Professional Help to Heal from Post Childhood Adversity Syndrome

187 *There are, says Kornfield, times when we need to get help:* These quotes are used with the permission of Jack Kornfield, PhD. Jack Kornfield, "Psychotherapy/Meditation: Even the Best Meditators Have Old Wounds to Heal" at http://buddhanet .net/psymed1.htm (accessed August 12, 2014).

187 *In this way, a therapist's unconditional acceptance:* Linda Graham, MFT, talks about this in a Clinical Conversation at the Community Institute for Psychotherapy in a talk titled "The Neuroscience of Attachment," first presented Fall 2008. You can find a transcript of her talk at http://lindagraham-mft.net/resources/pub lished-articles/the-neuroscience-of-attachment/ (accessed February 21, 20015).

187 *In one study, these changes remained in individuals:* J. Morath, M. Moreno-Villanueva, et al., "Effects of Psychotherapy on DNA Strand Break Accumulation Originating from Traumatic Stress," *Psychotherapy and Psychosomatics* 83, no. 5 (2014), 289–97.

187 *A fifty-eight-year-old patient of Dr. Vincent Felitti's:* These quotes are taken from a patient letter called "Dear Doctor: A Patient's Personal Case Study of Adverse Childhood Experiences," which appeared anonymously in *The Permanente Journal* 6, no. 1 (Winter 2002). This letter illustrates how health professionals often do not recognize the true, underlying basis for the problems they see, and how important the therapeutic process is in physical healing. You can read the entire letter here: http://www.acestudy.org/yahoo_site_admin/assets/docs/ Dear_Doctor.12893135.pdf (accessed February 24, 2015).

189 *Somatic Experiencing was developed by Peter A. Levine:* Peter Levine is author of the following books: with Maggie Kline, *Trauma-Proofing Your Kids: A Parents' Guide for Instilling Confidence, Joy and Resilience* (Berkeley, CA: North Atlantic Books, 2014);

with Maggie Phillips, *Freedom from Pain: Discover Your Body's Power to Overcome Physical Pain* (Louisville, CO: Sounds True, 2012); and *In an Unspoken Voice: How the Body Releases Trauma and Restores Goodness* (Berkeley, CA: North Atlantic Books, 2010).

192 *"Mental imagery is not the same thing"*: This understanding comes from my interview with Bernie Siegel, MD, on November 13, 2013, from email exchanges with him, and his book *The Art of Healing: Uncovering Your Inner Wisdom and Potential for Self-Healing* (Novato, CA: New World Library, 2013), 33. Siegel is also the author of *Love, Medicine & Miracles: Lessons Learned About Self-Healing from a Surgeon's Experience with Exceptional Patients* (New York: HarperCollins, 2011).

193 *If an individual practices a five-finger piano*: A. Pascual-Leone, D. Nguyet, L. G. Cohen, et al., "Modulation of Muscle Responses Evoked by Transcranial Magnetic Stimulation During the Acquisition of New Fine Motor Skills," *Journal of Neurophysiology* 74, no. 3 (September 1995), 1037–45.

193 *Even patients who took placebo pills*: S. Kam-Hansen, M. Jakubowski, J. M. Kelley, et al., "Altered Placebo and Drug Labeling Changes the Outcome of Episodic Migraine Attacks," *Science Translational Medicine* 6, no. 218 (January 8, 2014), 218ra5.

195 *I watched it float away*: Michele Rosenthal, *Before the World Intruded: Conquering the Past and Creating the Future* (Palm Beach Gardens, FL: Your Life After Trauma, LLC, 2012), 193–202.

198 *After a neurofeedback session, patients show*: Lanius recently conducted this study in which she and her colleagues gave individuals a single thirty-minute session of EEG Neurofeedback. They were able to help patients increase specific brain waves that elevated their sense of calmness. EEG Neurofeedback, however, is still a new modality, Lanius cautions. "But it is one more potential tool to add to the toolbox." R. C. Kluetsch, T. Ros, J. Théberge, P. A. Frewen, et al., "Plastic Modulation of PTSD Resting-State Networks and Subjective Wellbeing by EEG Neurofeedback," *ACTA Psychiatrica Scandinavica* 130, no. 2 (August 2014), 123–36, doi: 10.1111/acps.12229.

198 *By going through controlled exposure and reexposure*: For more on this, read Michael Specter, "Can Neuroscience Help Us Rewrite Our Most Traumatic Memories?," *The New Yorker* Dept. of Psychiatry, 46–47.

198 *"You will still know what happened"*: Researchers have been experimenting with how they might intervene in that "updating" process in order to separate our memory from the fear that we associate with it. Although researchers have long known how to induce fear, they have known far less about how to undo the relationship between a stimulus and a fear response. Daniela Schiller, PhD, assistant professor of neuroscience and psychiatry at Mount Sinai, has been working on ways to disentangle painful emotions from memories. She has found that after exposing individuals to an object that triggers deep fear, she can help them to have no negative emotions associated with it. She trained participants in a study to feel afraid when they saw a colored square by giving them a shock each time they viewed it. A day later, individuals were exposed to the squares again. Just the sight of the colored square caused them to show fear. Ten minutes later, Schiller showed one-third of the study participants the squares many more times—but without shocking them. She showed another group of people the squares without shocks several *hours* after reexposing them. The group that saw the square ten minutes

later without any shocks forgot their fear completely. The other group who was reexposed to the square hours later remained just as stress-reactive and frightened. You can read more about Schiller's work in the article by Michael Specter, "Can Neuroscience Help Us Rewrite Our Most Traumatic Memories?" *The New Yorker* Dept. of Psychiatry, 46–47. Also see D. Schiller, M. H. Monfils, C. M. Raio, et al., "Preventing the Return of Fear in Humans Using Reconsolidation Update Mechanisms," *Nature*, 463, no. 7277 (January 7, 2010), 49–53.

198 *EMDR therapy was developed by Francine Shapiro:* My understanding of EMDR is based on an interview I did with Francine Shapiro, PhD, on November 15, 2013, as well as on our follow-up emails. For more on EMDR therapy, read her *Getting Past Your Past: Take Control of Your Life with Self-Help Techniques from EMDR Therapy* (New York: Rodale, 2012).

200 *Shapiro found that she could help patients:* Shapiro points out that EMDR involves an eight-step process in order to help patients tap into negative emotions, and reprocess early memories. For more information on these eight steps, see Francine Shapiro's *Getting Past Your Past: Take Control of Your Life with Self-Help Techniques from EMDR Therapy* (New York: Rodale, 2012).

201 *EMDR therapy appears to link into the same neurological processes:* Recently, scientists at the University of Rochester were able to show that during sleep the brain does a "brainwash." As we sleep, cerebrospinal fluid washes through the brain, literally cleaning out harmful toxins and waste proteins that build up between brain cells during our waking hours, especially as we go through stressful events. Indeed, it's only during sleep that cerebrospinal fluid gets redirected deeper into our brain tissue, really cleaning out toxins. Researchers liken this process to "a dishwasher" in the brain. They found that during sleep, the system that circulates cerebrospinal fluid through the brain and nervous system pumps fluid into the brain and removes fluid at a very rapid pace. But once we are awake, the flow between cells slows to a trickle, like "closing a faucet." This removing of the gunk and junk in the brain appears to include removing the beta-amyloid concentrations that also increase while a person is awake, and decrease when we sleep—and that lead to the buildup of amyloid plaque, which contributes to Alzheimer's disease.

Other research shows that when we aren't getting adequate sleep or deep sleep, neurons in an area of the brain, the locus coeruleus, which is involved in how well we mediate the stress response, stop functioning properly.

L. Xie, H. Kang, W. Xu, et al., "Sleep Drives Metabolite Clearance from the Adult Brain," *Science* 342, no. 6156 (October 18, 2013), 373–77. You can read more about this research at http://www.npr.org/blogs/health/2013/10/18/236211811/brains-sweep-themselves-clean-of-toxins-during-sleep (accessed August 22, 2014) and http://thekojonnamdishow.org/shows/2014-08-18/science-sleep/transcript (accessed August 26, 2014).

201 *This integration can, in turn, lead to a reduction:* This study was done by Robert Stickgold, PhD, in the Department of Psychiatry at Harvard Medical School. R. Stickgold, "EMDR: A Putative Neurobiological Mechanism of Action," *Journal of Clinical Psychology* 58, no. 1 (January 2002), 61–75.

202 *But most things I was trying weren't really getting:* Priscilla's quotes come from a

series of phone interviews I did with her as well as from her writings in *Learning to Breathe: My Yearlong Quest to Bring Calm to My Life* (New York: Free Press, 2011).

Chapter Eight: Parenting Well When You Haven't Been Well Parented: Fourteen Strategies to Help You Help Your Children

205 *Even when a parent is stressed, if things settle down:* Robin Karr-Morse, coauthor of *Scared Sick: The Role of Childhood Trauma in Adult Disease*, spoke about this in this interview, Thomas Rogers, "How Stress Is Really Hurting Our Kids," *Salon* (January 2, 2012), http://www.salon.com/2012/01/02/how_stress_is_really_hurt ing_our_kids/ (accessed February 22, 2015) as well as in email exchanges with me on January 26–28, 2015.

205 *Even rats who inherited stress biomarker:* Inna Gaisler-Salomon, PhD, "Inheriting Stress," *New York Times*, March 7, 2014, http://www.nytimes.com/2014/03/09/ opinion/sunday/can-children-inherit-stress.html?_r=0 (accessed April 26, 2014).

205 *Similarly, when a human parent suffers:* J. G. Johnson, P. Cohen, S. Kasen, et al., "Association of Maladaptive Parental Behavior with Psychiatric Disorder Among Parents and Their Offspring," *Archives of General Psychiatry* 58, no. 5 (May 2001), 453–60.

207 *You can move from historic insecurity:* Daniel J. Siegel, MD, *Brainstorm: The Power and Purpose of the Teenage Brain* (New York: Penguin, 2014), 36.

208 *"Or more precisely, we need to help him learn":* Paul Tough, *How Children Succeed: Grit, Curiosity, and the Hidden Power of Character* (New York: First Mariner Books, 2013), 183.

208 *You lend support while supporting separation:* This understanding emerges from an interview with Daniel J. Siegel, MD, on October 16, 2015, as well as our email exchanges and material from his book *Brainstorm*, 33–34.

209 *"What are your options?":* Some of the suggestions in this chapter on how to speak to children in ways that encourage a sense of resiliency are loosely derived from Chick Moorman's book *Parent Talk: How to Talk to Your Children in Language that Builds Self-Esteem and Encourages Responsibility* (New York: Simon & Schuster, 1998).

210 *"Let your child be seen, be safe, be soothed:* Siegel, *Brainstorm*, 33–34.

210 *One way that we can be a calming, soothing:* Stephen W. Porges, PhD, *The Polyvagal Theory: Neurophysiological Foundations of Emotions, Attachment, Communication, and Self-Regulation* (New York: Norton, 2011).

210 *When we increase the activity of our child's vagus nerve:* Stephen Porges, PhD, explained in a recent talk at Saybrook University, Oakland, CA, https://www. saybrook.edu/forum/mbm/dr-stephen-porges-expert-heart-rate-variability-pro vides-address-venice-italy-evolutionary-and-p (accessed February 24, 2015): "The look of love is in your eyes. The look your heart can't disguise. The look of love is saying so much more, than just words can ever say." It is that face-to-face encounter, the look of love, which facilitates adaptive social engagement, and helps individuals to heal from trauma.

211 *We seek connection with them, we want to engage:* My understanding of the neurobiology of attachment and the role of the vagal nerve was helped greatly by the following essay by Linda Graham, MFT, who talks about this in a Clinical Conversation at the Community Institute for Psychotherapy in a talk titled "The Neuroscience of Attachment," first presented Fall 2008. You can find a transcript

of her talk at http://lindagraham-mft.net/resources/published-articles/the-neuroscience-of-attachment/ (accessed February 21, 2015).

212 *Recent science on memory and adversity confirms*: D. Schiller, M. H. Monfils, C. M. Raio, et al., "Preventing the Return of Fear in Humans Using Reconsolidation Update Mechanisms," *Nature* 63, no. 7277 (January 7, 2010), 49–53.

213 *"That sounds hard"*: Krissy Pozatek, LCSW, writes about this in her article, "How to Raise a Resilient Child," (December 12, 2014), http://www.mindbodygreen.com/0-16635/how-to-raise-a-resilient-child.html. Pozatek is the author of *Brave Parenting: A Buddhist-Inspired Guide to Raising Emotionally Resilient Children* (Somerville, MA: Wisdom Publications, 2014).

213 *You can send two messages at once*: Ibid.

214 *According to neuropsychologist Rick Hanson, PhD*: Rick Hanson, PhD, is Senior Fellow of the Greater Good Science Center and author of *Hardwiring Happiness: The New Brain Science of Contentment, Calm, and Confidence* (New York: Harmony, 2013; Oakland, CA: New Harbinger, 2009).

214 *Researcher John Gottman, MD, PhD*: John Gottman, MD, PhD, talks about this 5-to-1 ratio of positive to negative interactions in this talk, available on YouTube: "The Magic Relationship Ratio," https://www.youtube.com/watch?v=X-w9SE315GtA (accessed February 25, 2015).

216 *Which means we "have to build stop signs"*: Brother David Steindl-Rast, a Benedictine monk, talks about "the gentle power" of gratefulness in this TED talk: https://www.ted.com/talks/david_steindl_rast_want_to_be_happy_be_grateful (accessed August 19, 2014).

216 *Matthew Lieberman, PhD, professor of psychology*: J. D. Creswell, B. M. Way, M. D. Lieberman, et al., "Neural Correlates of Dispositional Mindfulness During Affect Labeling," *Psychosomatic Medicine* 69, no. 6 (July–August 2007), 560–65; L. J. Burklund, J. D. Creswell, M. D. Lieberman, et al., "The Common and Distinct Neural Bases of Affect Labeling and Reappraisal in Healthy Adults," *Frontiers in Psychology* 5 (March 24, 2014), 221.

220 *They lack "consistent, protective, reliable"*: These quotes are taken from a transcript from The Forum at Harvard School of Public Health titled, "The Toxic Stress of Early Childhood Adversity: Rethinking Health and Education Policy," February 7, 2012, http://developingchild.harvard.edu/resources/multimedia/lectures_and_presentations/hsph-forum/ (accessed February 20, 2015).

221 *But kids need to have other nonparental adults around*: Dan Siegel, MD, talked about this in his appearance on the *Diane Rehm Show* on January 6, 2014, http://thedianerehmshow.org/shows/2014-01-06/daniel-siegel-brainstorm-power-and-purpose-teenage-brain (accessed August 10, 2014).

221 *Mentoring groups suggest that young people receive support*: Search Institute, "40 Developmental Assets for Adolescents," http://www.search-institute.org/content/40-developmental-assets-adolescents-ages-12-18 (accessed February 24, 2015).

223 *American teenagers cite their stress level as being*: You can read more in this press release: "American Psychological Association Survey Shows Teen Stress Rivals That of Adults" (February 11, 2014), http://www.apa.org/news/press/releases/2014/02/teen-stress.aspx (accessed May 19, 2014).

224 *One of the conference leaders, Jack Kornfield, PhD:* The Mindfulness in Education Conference: Bringing Mindfulness Practice to Children Grades K–12 was held July 25 to 27, 2014, at the OMEGA Institute, Rhinebeck, New York.

224 *One study found that students who take a ten-minute lesson:* Jonah Lehrer, "Under Pressure: The Search for a Stress Vaccine," *Wired* (July 28, 2010), http://www .wired.com/magazine/2010/07/ff_stress_cure/all/1 (accessed August 9, 2014). In this article Lehrer reports on a 2010 study led by Sian Beilock, a psychologist at the University of Chicago, who found that a ten-minute lesson in mindfulness meditation seemed to reduce stress in those taking a high-stakes math exam, leading to a five-point increase on average.

224 *Individuals trained in meditation perform:* R. Prakash, I. Dubey, P. Abhishek, et al., "Long-term Vihangam Yoga Meditation and Scores on Tests of Attention," *Perceptual Motor Skills* 110, no. 3, part 2 (June 2010), 1139–48; F. A. Huppert and D. M. Johnson, "A Controlled Trial of Mindfulness Training in Schools; The Importance of Practice for an Impact on Well-being," *Journal of Positive Psychology* 5, no. 4 (July 2010), 264–74. See more at http://mindfulnessinschools.org (accessed August 9, 2014).

224 *Another study found that adolescents who took a course on mindfulness:* W. Kuyken, K. Weare, O. C. Ukoumunne, et al., "Effectiveness of the Mindfulness in Schools Programme: Non-Randomised Controlled Feasibility Study," *British Journal of Psychiatry* 203, no. 2 (August 2013), 126–31.

224 *Christina Bethell, PhD, professor at the Johns Hopkins Bloomberg School of Public Health:* C. D. Bethell, P. Newacheck, E. Hawes, et al. Adverse Childhood Experiences: Assessing the Impact on Health and School Engagement and the Mitigating Role of Resilience. *Health Affairs*, 33, no. 12 (2014): 2106–15.

225 *Working with more than two thousand teachers and staff:* R. C. Whitaker, T. Dearth-Wesley, R. A. Gooze, et al., "Adverse Childhood Experiences, Dispositional Mindfulness, and Adult Health," *Preventive Medicine* 67 (October 2014), 47–53.

In Conclusion

228 *Indeed, it is "our misfortunes that drive":* These quotes emerge from writer Andrew Solomon's TED Talk "How the Worst Moments in Our Lives Make Us Who We Are" (filmed March 2014) and were honed through email exchanges with Solomon. The TED talk can be found at http://www.ted.com/talks/andrew_sol omon_how_the_worst_moments_in_our_lives_make_us_who_we_are?lan guage=en (accessed February 24, 2015).

228 *Researchers have found that in the last decades:* Chioun Lee, "Childhood Abuse and Elevated Markers of Inflammation in Adulthood: Do the Effects Differ Across Life Course Stages?," http://paa2013.princeton.edu/papers/130463 (accessed February 24, 2015) and Chioun Lee, "Childhood Abuse and Physiological Dysregulation in Midlife and Old Age," http://dx.doi.org/doi:10.7282/T39W0D8D (accessed February 24, 2015).

228 *People who met up with adversity in the past:* C. Croft, E. W. Dunn, and J. Quoidbach, "From Tribulations to Appreciation: Experiencing Adversity in the Past Predicts Greater Savoring in the Present," *Social Psychological and Personality Science* (November 25, 2013).

228 *It has been said that if child abuse and neglect were:* This quote is attributed to psychologist John Briere, PhD, who has observed that if child abuse and neglect were to disappear, the *Diagnostic and Statistical Manual*—an 886-page tome cataloging some three hundred mental disorders—would shrink to the size of a pamphlet, and the prisons would empty in two generations. Claudia Rowe, "Fostering Resilience," *Crosscut* (July 24, 2013), http://crosscut.com/2013/07/resilience-in-foster-kids/ (accessed February 24, 2015).

229 *In one recent study of 125,000 patients:* V. J. Felitti and R. F. Anda, "The Lifelong Effects of Adverse Childhood Experiences," in Chadwick's *Child Maltreatment: Sexual Abuse and Psychological Maltreatment,* vol. 2, edited by D. L. Chadwick, A. P. Giardino, R. Alexander, et al., (MO: St. Louis), STM Learning, 2014, 211–12.

230 *But as health-care dollars have become stretched:* Roni Caryn Rabin, "15-Minute Visits Take a Toll on the Doctor-Patient Relationship," *Kaiser Health News* (April 21, 2014), http://www.kaiserhealthnews.org/stories/2014/april/21/15-minute-doctor-visits.aspx (accessed August 10, 2014).

231 *According to the Centers for Disease Control:* Centers for Disease Control and Prevention, "Child Abuse and Neglect Cost the United States $124 Billion," http://www.cdc.gov/media/releases/2012/p0201_child_abuse.html (accessed August 29, 2014).

231 *The lifetime health-care cost for each individual:* Ibid.

231 *Dr. Jeffrey Brenner, a 2013 MacArthur Foundation genius:* Jeffrey Brenner, MD, is founder and executive director of the Camden Coalition of Healthcare Providers and a 2013 MacArthur Foundation genius award winner. He did groundbreaking work in Camden, New Jersey, by using data to identify people who were hospital emergency room "frequent fliers." Often they are the same people who have suffered from Adverse Childhood Experiences. Brenner is the medical director of the Urban Health Institute at Cooper University Healthcare. Read his essay about ACEs at Jeffrey Brenner MD, "The Secret to Better Care: It Really Is All in Your Head," Philly.com (January 29, 2014), http://www.philly.com/philly/blogs/fieldclinic/The-Secret-to-Better-Care-It-Really-Is-All-in-Your-Head.html (accessed February 25, 2015).

232 *"Now you have both a science-based imperative and a moral responsibility":* Iris Adler, "How Childhood Neglect Harms the Brain," *CommonHealth* (June 26, 2014), http://commonhealth.wbur.org/2014/06/trauma-abuse-brain-matters (accessed August 7, 2014).

232 *Robert W. Block, MD, past president of AAP:* This focus group featured talks by a group of leading experts, including Robert W. Block, MD, and was titled "The Toxic Stress of Early Childhood Adversity: Rethinking Health and Education," February 7, 2012, in Boston, http://developingchild.harvard.edu/resources/multimedia/lectures_and_presentations/hsph-forum/ (accessed May 20, 2014). See also B. M. Kuehn, "AAP: Toxic Stress Threatens Kids' Long-term Health," *JAMA* 312, no. 6 (August 2014), 585–86.

233 *We're leaving a lot of children behind:* This understanding comes from my email conversations with Robin Karr-Morse as well as from this interview: Thomas Rogers, "How Stress Is Really Hurting Our Kids, *Salon* (January 2, 2012), http://www.salon.com/2012/01/02/how_stress_is_really_hurting_our_kids/ (accessed May 15, 2014).

RESOURCES AND FURTHER READING

Tara Brach, PhD, *True Refuge: Finding Peace and Freedom in Your Own Awakened Heart* (New York: Bantam, 2013), and *Radical Acceptance: Embracing Your Life with the Heart of a Buddha* (New York: Bantam, 2003).

Richard Davidson, PhD, *The Emotional Life of Your Brain: How Its Unique Patterns Affect the Way You Think, Feel, and Live—and How You Can Change Them* (New York: Penguin, 2012).

James S. Gordon, MD, *Unstuck: Your Guide to the Seven-Stage Journey Out of Depression* (New York: Penguin, 2008).

Rick Hanson, PhD, *Hardwiring Happiness: The New Brain Science of Contentment, Calm, and Confidence* (New York: Harmony, 2013); *Just One Thing: Developing a Buddha Brain One Simple Practice at a Time* (Oakland, CA: New Harbinger, 2011); and *Buddha's Brain: The Practical Neuroscience of Happiness, Love, and Wisdom* (Oakland, CA: New Harbinger, 2009).

Robin Karr-Morse and Meredith S. Wiley, *Ghosts in the Nursery: Tracing the Roots of Violence* (New York: Grove Press, 2013), and *Scared Sick: The Role of Childhood Trauma in Adult Disease* (New York: Basic Books, 2012).

Jack Kornfield, PhD, *A Lamp in the Darkness: Illuminating the Path Through Difficult Times* (Louisville, CO: Sounds True, 2014), and *The Wise Heart: A Guide to the Universal Teachings of Buddhist Psychology* (New York: Bantam 2009).

Jack Kornfield, PhD, and Daniel J. Siegel, MD, *Bringing Home the Dharma: Awakening Right Where You Are* (Boston, MA: Shambhala, 2012).

Peter A. Levine, PhD, and Maggie Kline, *Trauma-Proofing Your Kids: A Parents' Guide for Instilling Confidence, Joy and Resilience* (Berkeley, CA: North Atlantic Books, 2014).

Peter A. Levine, PhD, and Gabor Mate, *In an Unspoken Voice: How the Body Releases Trauma and Restores Goodness* (Berkeley, CA: North Atlantic Books, 2010).

Peter A. Levine, PhD, and Maggie Phillips, *Freedom from Pain: Discover Your Body's Power to Overcome Physical Pain* (Louisville, CO: Sounds True, 2012).

Kelly McGonigal, PhD, *The Upside of Stress: Why Stress Is Good for You, and How to Get Good at It* (New York: Avery, 2015), and *The Willpower Instinct: How Self-Control Works, Why It Matters, and What You Can Do to Get More of It* (New York: Avery, 2013).

James W. Pennebaker, PhD, *Writing to Heal: A Guided Journal for Recovering from Trauma and Emotional Upheaval* (Oakland, CA: New Harbinger Publications, 2004).

Stephen W. Porges, PhD, *The Polyvagal Theory: Neurophysiological Foundations of Emotions, Attachment, Communication, and Self-Regulation* (New York: Norton, 2011).

Krissy Pozatek, *Brave Parenting: A Buddhist-Inspired Guide to Raising Emotionally Resilient Children* (Somerville, MA: Wisdom Publications, 2014).

Francine Shapiro, PhD, *Getting Past Your Past: Take Control of Your Life with Self-Help Techniques from EMDR Therapy* (New York: Rodale, 2012).

Bernie S. Siegel, MD, *The Art of Healing: Uncovering Your Inner Wisdom and Potential for Self-Healing* (Novato, CA: New World Library, 2013) and *Love, Medicine & Miracles: Lessons Learned About Self-Healing from a Surgeon's Experience with Exceptional Patients* (New York: HarperCollins, 2011).

Daniel J. Siegel, MD, *Brainstorm: The Power and Purpose of the Teenage Brain* (New York: Penguin, 2014), and *Mindsight: The New Science of Personal Transformation* (New York: Bantam, 2010).

Daniel J. Siegel, MD, and Tina Payne Bryson, *No-Drama Discipline: The Whole-Brain Way to Calm the Chaos and Nurture Your Child's Developing Mind* (New York: Bantam, 2014), and *The Whole-Brain Child: 12 Revolutionary Strategies to Nurture Your Child's Developing Mind* (New York: Bantam, 2012).

Andrew Solomon, *Far from the Tree: Parents, Children, and the Search for Identity* (New York: Scribner, 2013) and *The Noonday Demon: An Atlas of Depression* (New York: Scribner, 2002).

Paul Tough, *How Children Succeed: Grit, Curiosity, and the Hidden Power of Character* (New York: Mariner, 2013).

Bessel van der Kolk, MD, *The Body Keeps the Score: Brain, Mind, and Body in the Healing of Trauma* (New York: Viking, 2014).

Priscilla Warner, *Learning to Breathe: My Yearlong Quest to Bring Calm to My Life* (New York: Free Press, 2011).

INDEX

A
Abeles, Vicki, 132
abuse, 111
  emotional, 16, 48, 72, 111
  physical, 16, 25, 72, 108, 111
  sexual, *see* sexual abuse
Academy of American Pediatrics (AAP),
  232
ACEsConnection.com, 225, 234
ACEsTooHigh.com, 225, 234
achievement-obsessed culture, 132
addiction, 47, 54, 72, 149
  alcoholism, 15, 25, 47
  in parent, 25, 31
Addison's disease, 62
ADHD, 109, 131
adolescence, *see* puberty and adolescence
adrenal-hypothalamus-pituitary stress axis,
  29–32, 76, 124, 211
adrenaline, 29, 46, 84
Adverse Childhood Experiences (ACE),
  xiv–xix, 9–10, 63–65, 131, 150,
  227–34
  healing from, *see* healing journey
  normal childhood challenges vs., xvii,
    207–9
  parenting by people with, 115–21
  secrecy and shame associated with,
    67–68, 71, 151, 217
  societal awareness of, 153
  in women vs. men, 96
Adverse Childhood Experiences, research
  on, 24–27, 28, 97–100, 229, 231
  by Anda, 12–16, 25, 27, 41, 47–48, 96,
    97, 99, 100, 111, 242–43n

by Fairweather, 97–100
by Felitti, 10–16, 25, 27, 41, 47–48, 96,
  97, 99, 100, 111, 113, 151–53, 242n
Adverse Childhood Experiences Score,
  xxiv, 13–15, 32, 43, 48, 49, 113,
  151, 152, 157, 231–32
  allostatic load and, 61
  of author, xvi
  autoimmune disease and, 98–99
  of Georgia, 23
  of John, 23
  of Kat, 22
  of Kendall, 96, 99
  of Laura, 23
  in men, 104
  in women, 104
Adverse Childhood Experiences Survey,
  xvi, 12–15, 16, 25, 32, 122, 229–30,
  242n
  humiliation question in, 47
  questions to ask yourself about, 152
  taking the survey, xxi–xxiv, 151–53
adversity, 209, 227–28
  childhood challenges that foster
    resilience, xvii, 207–9
  context and, 220
  inheritance of, xix, 145, 201, 219–20
  lack of, 63–65
  upside to, 64–65
aging, 16
alcoholism, 15, 47
  of parent, 25
alertness and hypervigilance, 39–40, 57,
  106, 123
Alice, 187–88

allostatic load, 61, 76
alopecia areata, 56
Alzheimer's disease, 51, 262n
American Psychological Association, 132
amygdala, 49, 56, 84, 87, 105, 107, 108,
    123, 133, 134, 141, 177, 201, 211,
    217
amyloid plaque, 262n
Anda, Robert, 12–16, 25, 27, 41, 47–48,
    96, 97, 99, 100, 111, 242–43n
anger, 140, 143, 158
    somatic exercises and, 192
Anna Karenina (Tolstoy), 28
antibodies, 101, 102
antiphospholipid syndrome, 100
anxiety, 47, 51, 52, 54, 56, 57, 64, 78, 82,
    87, 104, 107, 109, 112, 125, 128,
    141
    in children and teens, 130, 131, 132
    GABA and, 178
    in parents, 127–28
    somatic exercises and, 192
    in women, 96, 104, 107
apologizing, 211–12
art therapy, 160
asthma, 32, 37
    Stephen's experience with, 55
attachment, 141–43, 145–46, 207, 211,
    217, 256n
    four S's of, 210
August: Osage County (Letts), 145
autism, 124
autoantibodies, 101, 102
autoimmune diseases, xiii, xvii, 14, 37, 38
    ACE Scores and, 98–99
    Ellie's experience with, 41, 183
    Harriet's experience with, 73–74
    Kendall's experience with, 94–96,
        99
    Kennedy's experience with, 62
    Mary's experience with, 44, 45, 179
    in men, 98, 103, 104
    in women, 96–104, 112–13
    see also specific conditions

B
babies, see infants
back pain, 63–64, 65, 97
bacteria, 30, 101
    gut, 181–84
baggage, managing, 207

Before the World Intruded: Conquering
    the Past and Creating the Future
    (Rosenthal), 196
Beilock, Sian, 265n
beliefs, negative, 199–200
Bercelli, David, 178
Bethell, Christina, 131, 224
bipolar disorder, 47, 54
blame, xviii, xix, 106
Block, Robert W., 232
Blumberg, Hilary P., 107–9
body, 177–81
    body work and, 179–81
    tai chi and qigong and, 169–70
    Trauma Release Exercises and, 178–79
    yoga and, 177–78, 179
Body Keeps the Score, The: Brain, Mind, and
    Body in the Healing of Trauma (van
    der Kolk), 103–4
Boorstein, Sylvia, 169
boundaries, 139
bowel disorders, 97, 181–82
    irritable bowel syndrome, 32, 34, 37, 96
Brach, Tara, 163, 164, 169
brain, xv, 10, 25, 49
    adolescence and, 52–54
    adversity's effects on shape and size of, 49
    amygdala in, 49, 56, 84, 87, 105, 107, 108,
        123, 133, 134, 141, 177, 201, 211, 217
    in babies, 123
    in boys, 108–9
    chronic unpredictable stress and, 41–43
    corpus callosum in, 53
    default mode network of, 137–38, 140
    development of, 24, 26, 27, 35, 36, 41,
        46, 50, 66, 75, 76, 101, 109, 123,
        141–42, 205–6
    fear and, 110
    frontal lobe in, 107, 161, 177
    GABA and, 177–78, 182, 217
    in girls, 104–9
    gray matter in, 49, 51, 108, 162, 171
    guided imagery and, 192, 193
    gut and, 181–84
    hippocampus in, 42, 49, 51–53, 56, 84,
        105–7, 108, 110, 161, 162, 201
    hypothalamus in, 29–32
    inflammation in, 50–52, 56–58, 61, 66,
        78, 110
    information processing center in, 200–201
    insula in, 108, 140

memories and, 83–84
microglia in, 50–52, 57
and naming emotions, 216
negativity bias of, 214
neurofeedback and, 197–98
neuron creation in, 112, 151, 171, 172, 206
neuron pruning in, 50–54, 56, 57, 109, 162
plasticity of, xix, 58, 75, 80, 150
prefrontal cortex in, 49, 53, 105–7, 108, 177, 211
rebooting, 150
relationships and, 136, 137, 142, 145–46
reset tone in, 50–52, 57
reversing damage to, 58–59
scans of, 49, 105, 127, 130, 137, 140, 161
stress and, 28, 29, 35–36, 122–23
synaptic connections in, 24, 51, 52, 57, 84, 142, 151, 171, 172, 206
therapy and, 187
toxic stress and, 66–67
two sides of, 192–93
washing of, during sleep, 262n
white matter in, 49, 51, 171
yoga and, 177–78
Brainstorm: The Power and Purpose of the Teenage Brain (Siegel), 138
breathing, 162–63, 189, 190
Brenner, Jeffrey, 231–32, 266n
Briere, John, 266n
Briggs, Katherine Cook, 24
Brown University, 16
Buddhism, 85, 87, 164, 168, 174
bullying, 129–31, 134, 223

C

cancer, 14, 16, 32, 37–38
cardiovascular disease, 15, 16, 37–38, 114, 115, 130, 132
    broken heart syndrome, 31, 32
    heart attack, 31
    Laura's experience with, 5, 23, 32, 40
    stroke, 16, 32
Carnegie Mellon University, 158
celiac disease, 94, 95, 96, 159, 183
Center for Mind-Body Medicine, 175
Center for Mindfulness in Medicine, Health Care and Society, 168

Center for Neurobiology of Stress, 182
Center on Healthy, Resilient Children, 232
Center on the Developing Child, 66, 72, 232
Centers for Disease Control and Prevention (CDC), 10, 11–12, 97, 231, 242n
    challenges that foster resilience, xvii, 207–9
Chekhov, Anton, 145
Child and Adolescent Research and Education (CARE), 36
Child Emotion Laboratory, 36
Childhood Trauma Questionnaire (CTQ), 26
Chodron, Pema, 169
cholesterol, 15
chromosomes, 35
chronic fatigue syndrome (CFS; myalgic encephalomyelitis; ME), 16, 32, 34, 37, 56–57, 96, 97
Chronic Unpredictable Toxic Stress (CUTS), 67–68, 82, 84, 97, 113, 122, 145, 150, 174, 201, 204, 216
    childhood challenges that foster resilience vs., xvii, 207–9
Cindy, 115–19, 218–19, 222
Colelli, Gina, 202
college, 132, 133, 134
compassion, 171, 172–74
connection, 184–85
contagious emotions, 125–27
Copeland, William E., 130
coping mechanisms, 15
Core Energetic massage, 180, 181
corpus callosum, 53
cortisol, 29, 30, 36, 38, 46, 77, 100–101, 112, 124, 133, 161
Cozolino, Louis, 145
cranialsacral work, 180
C-reactive protein (CRP), 130
creative visualization, 192–94, 195
cytokines, 30, 31

D

David and Goliath (Gladwell), 62
Davidson, Richard, 258n
death:
    of child, 31
    of grandparent, 64, 66
    of parent, 16, 31, 48, 62–63, 138, 139
    risk of, 81
    of sibling, 31

depression, 14–15, 16, 47–49, 51, 52, 54,
    56, 57, 64, 76, 80, 109, 149, 224,
    248n
  in children and teens, 130, 131, 132
  GABA and, 178
  genes and, 110–12
  in men, 48, 104, 110–12
  of parent, 25, 31, 48, 127–28
  in women, 48, 96, 97, 104, 107, 110–13
Developmental Trauma Disorder, 150
Dharma Brothers, 164
diabetes, 15, 16, 32, 38
*Diagnostic and Statistical Manual of Mental
    Disorders,* 150, 228
diet, 182–84
disease, xv, 15, 27, 30–32, 81, 149
  autoimmune, *see* autoimmune diseases
  correlation between types of Adverse
    Childhood Experiences and types
    of, 16
  multifactorial nature of, xvii–xviii
  parental closeness and, 114–15
  telomeres and, 16
  see also specific conditions
divorce, 16, 31, 32, 138, 224
DNA, 35, 36, 125
  telomeres and, 16
  therapy and, 187
Dobbs, David, 251n
doctors, 152–53, 229–31
drawing, 160
Duke University, 16, 77, 130

E
eating disorders, 54
Electroencephalographic (EEG)
    Neurofeedback, 197–98
Eliot, T. S., 27
Ellie, 40–41, 46
  autoimmune condition of, 41, 183
  diet and, 183
  mindfulness meditation and, 167–68
EMDR (Eye Movement Desensitization
    and Reprocessing), 198–201
Emory University, 74
emotional abuse, 16, 48, 72, 111
emotional neglect, 31, 108
emotional resilience, *see* resilience
emotions:
  awareness of, 171–72
  contagious, 125–27

disassociation from, 138–40, 141
  Eye Movement Desensitization and
    Reprocessing and, 198–201
  good, amplifying, 213–15
  memories and, 198–99, 261n
  mindfulness and, 162
  naming of, 216–17
  painful, 157, 198
  physicality of, 29
  positive, 139
  regulation of, 140–41
  repression of, 157–58
  validating and normalizing, 212–13
  writing down, 157–58
empathic stress, 125
empathy, 171, 228
endocrine function, 37
epigenetics, 35–38, 57–59, 103, 246n
Epstein-Barr virus, 34
estrogen, 100–102
eye gaze, 210–11
Eye Movement Desensitization and
    Reprocessing (EMDR), 198–201

F
Fairweather, DeLisa, 97–102
falls, 31
*Far from the Tree: Parents, Children, and the
    Search for Identity* (Solomon), 227
fatigue, 128
fear, 31, 39, 57, 87, 107, 141, 143, 261n
  amygdala and, 49, 105, 107, 211
  brain and, 110
  fight-or-flight response and, 29, 36, 87,
    101, 105, 128, 138, 178
  memory and, 198
Felitti, Vincent J., 10–16, 25, 27, 41, 47–48,
    96, 97, 99, 100, 111, 113, 151–53,
    158, 187, 229–30, 241–42nn
fibroid tumors, 37, 74
fibromyalgia, 37, 96, 97
fight-or-flight response, 29, 36, 87, 101,
    105, 128, 138, 178
financial problems, 31
Fischer, Norman, 169
foods, 182–84
forgiveness, 173, 174–77, 195
Four Quartets (Eliot), 27
four S's, 210
freeze state, 123, 188, 189
Freudian theory, 24

G

GABA (gamma-aminobutyric acid), 177–78, 182, 217
gender, *see* men: women
genemethylation, 35
genes, xv, 124
  CRHR1, 110–12
  epigenetics and, 35–38, 57–59, 103, 246n
  5-HTTLPR, 75–77
  as link between childhood adversity and adult depression, 110–12
  NR3C1, 77
  sensitivity, 75–78, 80–81
  stress and, 75–78
  stress vulnerability, 77–78, 80
  variants (alleles) of, 250n
  see also DNA
Georgia, 8–9, 10, 21, 23, 41, 46, 78–81, 83, 212
  ACE Score of, 23
  illnesses of, 9
  intergenerational trauma and, 219–20
  relationships of, 79
  somatic experiencing and, 190–91
Ghosts from the Nursery: Tracing the Roots of Violence (Karr-Morse and Wiley), 123
Gladwell, Malcolm, 62, 63
glucocorticoids (GCs), 100–102
Goldfinch, The (Tartt), 145
Gordon, James, 175–76
Gottman, John, 214
Grace, 119–21, 128
Graham, Alice, 127
Graham, Linda, 260n
gratitude, 216
Graves' disease, 73–74
guided imagery, 192–94
Guillain-Barré syndrome, xiii–xiv
guilt, 141
gut health, 181–84

H

Hanson, Rick, 214–15
Harriet, 72–74, 83, 85, 86
  Grave's disease of, 73–74
Harvard University, 60, 66, 88, 114–15
  Center on the Developing Child, 66, 72, 232
Hashimoto's thyroiditis, 100
headaches, 16, 32, 128
  migraines, 37, 97, 133

Head Start, 24, 225
healing journey, 149–85
  body in, 177–81
  body work in, 179–81
  connection in, 184–85
  drawing in, 160
  forgiveness in, 173, 174–77
  gut health in, 181–84
  loving-kindness in, 172–74, 175
  meditation in, *see* meditation
  Mindsight in, 170–72
  professional help in, *see* professional help
  resilience score in, 154–57
  tai chi and qigong in, 169–70
  taking the Adverse Childhood Experiences Survey, xxi–xxiv, 151–53
  Trauma Release Exercises in, 178–79
  writing in, 157–60
  yoga in, 177–78, 179
health care:
  costs of, 231
  medical trauma and, 31, 32–34
  pediatric, 232–33
  practitioners in, 152–53, 229–31
heart disease, *see* cardiovascular disease
Herringa, Ryan, 104–7, 161
high blood pressure (hypertension), 114, 115, 130
hippocampus, 42, 49, 51–53, 56, 84, 105–7, 108, 110, 161, 162, 201
hormones, 84, 125
  estrogen, 100–102
  oxytocin, 74, 82, 184–85, 217
  stress, *see* stress hormones
  testosterone, 103
How Children Succeed (Tough), 208
HPA (hypothalamus-pituitary-adrenal) stress axis, 29–32, 37, 38, 76, 124, 211
hugs, 217
humiliation and put-downs, 25, 31, 47, 68, 209
Hurley, Kat, 17–21, 23, 40, 41, 46, 68, 86, 159–60, 184
  ACE Score of, 22
  diet and, 183–84
  grandmother of, 19, 222–23
  immune system problems of, 20–21, 22
  mindfulness meditation and, 164–67
  relationships of, 142–43, 167
  writing of, 159

hypertension (high blood pressure), 114,
115, 130
hypervigilance and alertness, 39–40, 57,
106, 123
hypnosis, 193, 194–96
hypothalamus-pituitary-adrenal (HPA)
stress axis, 29–32, 76, 124, 211

I

Ibsen, Henrik, 145
illness, see disease
immune system, xvii–xviii, 10, 25, 29, 30,
35, 37, 38, 132, 158
incest survivors and, 104
infections and, 30
Kat's problems with, 20–21, 22
testosterone and, 103
incest, 104
infants, 123–24
brain of, 123
parents' stress and, 125–27
inflammation, xv, 10, 36, 37, 81, 149, 151,
161, 162
in brain, 50–52, 56–58, 61, 66, 78, 110
C-reactive protein and, 130
glucocorticoids and, 100–102
Kat's experience with, 20–21, 22
stress and, 29–32
insight, 170–71
Insight Meditation Group, 168
insula, 108, 140
integration, 171
interpersonal biology, 52
irritable bowel syndrome, 32, 34, 37, 96
*I Think I'll Make It: A True Story of Lost and
Found* (Hurley), 159

J

jail, 41
John, 5–7, 9, 10, 21, 23, 41, 46, 129, 145
ACE Score of, 23
bullying experience of, 129
diet and, 183
illnesses of, 6–7, 169
intergenerational trauma and, 220
relationships of, 7, 134–36, 143
reliable adult and, 222
tai chi and qigong practiced by, 169–70
Johns Hopkins medical institutions, xv,
115, 131, 224
Jungian theory, 24

K

Kaiser Permanente, 10–11, 12, 97, 241n,
242n
Karr-Morse, Robin, 123–24, 233
Kassam, Karim, 258n
Kat, see Hurley, Kat
Kaufman, Joan, 36, 37–38
Kendall, 89–96
ACE Score of, 96, 99
autoimmune disorders of, 94–96, 99
celiac disease of, 94, 95, 96, 159, 183
diet and, 183
document written by, 159
intergenerational trauma and, 219
obsessive-compulsive disorder of, 91,
93, 96
reliable adult and, 222
Kennedy, John F., 62
kindling, 123, 140
Kornfield, Jack, 169, 174–75, 177, 186–87,
224

L

Laliotis, Deany, 205–6
Lanius, Ruth, 137–41, 197, 199, 261n
Laura, 3–5, 9, 10, 21, 23, 32, 40, 41, 46, 68,
109, 149, 217–18
ACE Score of, 23
alertness of, 39–40
body work and, 181
guided imagery and, 193–94
health problems of, 5
heart disease of, 5, 23, 32, 40
leaders, 62
Learning to Breathe (Warner), 71
Letts, Tracy, 145
Levine, Peter A., 189, 190
Lieberman, Matthew, 216
limit-setting, 213
Lincoln, Abraham, 62
longevity, 15, 16
love, 143, 145–46
loving-kindness, 172–74, 175
loving yourself, 157
lung disease, 16, 32
lupus, 16, 32, 98, 99, 100, 102

M

magnetic resonance imaging (MRI), 49, 105
functional (fMRI), 127, 140
Magyari, Trish, 169

marriage of parents:
  discord in, 16
  divorce and, 16, 31, 32, 138, 224
Mary, 43–46, 212
  autoimmune condition of, 44, 45, 179
  body work and, 180–81
  reliable adult and, 222
  Trauma Release Exercises and, 178–79
Massage Rho, 180, 181
Mayer, Emeran, 182
McCarthy, Margaret, 34–36, 41–42, 46,
    50–52, 57–59, 102–3, 112
McClinn, Kate, 257n
McEwen, Bruce S., 61
McGonigal, Kelly, 81–82
medical care, see health care
Medical University of South Carolina, 112
medication, 162–63, 199
meditation, 172
  compassion, 172–74
  forgiveness, 175–77
  mindfulness, see mindfulness
    meditation
  moving, 169
  therapy and, 186–87
memory(ies), 83–87, 152
  brain and, 83–84
  consolidation and reconsolidation of,
    84–85, 88
  emotions and, 198–99, 261n
  explicit, 85–86, 152
  Eye Movement Desensitization and
    Reprocessing and, 198–201
  fear and, 198
  of good vs. bad interactions, 214
  implicit, 85–86, 152
  neuron growth and, 112
men:
  ACE Scores in, 104
  autoimmune diseases in, 98, 103, 104
  boys' brains and, 108–9
  childhood adversity in, 96
  depression in, 48, 104, 110–12
  physiological differences between
    women and, 100
  stress in, 103
mental imagery, 192–94
mentors, 74, 76, 80, 220–23
metabolic syndrome, 128
methyl groups, 36
metta, 173

Michele, see Rosenthal, Michele
microbiome, 181–84
microglia, 50–52, 57
migraines, 37, 97, 133
military service, 233
mindfulness-based stress reduction
    (MBSR), 161, 162, 168, 169
Mindfulness in Education Conference,
    223–24
mindfulness meditation, 161–69, 175, 190
  Ellie's experience with, 167–68
  Kat's experience with, 164–67
  in schools, 223–25
  vipassana, 164, 166, 168, 169
Mindsight, 170–72
miscarriage, 31, 101
Mood Disorders Research Program, 108
mood words, 139
multiple sclerosis (MS), 16, 31, 32, 100, 103
muscular tension, 178
myalgic encephalomyelitis, see chronic
    fatigue syndrome
Myers, Isabel Briggs, 24
Myss, Caroline, 244n

N
narcissism, 69–70
National Institute of Mental Health
    (NIMH), 47, 56
negative beliefs, 199–200
neglect, 16, 37–38, 68, 72
  emotional, 31, 108
nervous system, 162–63, 189, 190
neurofeedback, 197–98
neurogenic tremors, 178
neurons:
  creation of, 112, 151, 171, 172, 206
  pruning of, 50–54, 56, 57, 109, 162
  synaptic connections between, 24, 51,
    52, 57, 84, 142, 151, 171, 172, 206
Nhat Hanh, Thich, 87
Noonday Demon, The: An Atlas of
    Depression (Solomon), 227
nurturing mothers, 128–29
nutrition, 182–84

O
osteoporosis, 34
overweight and obesity, 11, 15, 38, 96, 128,
    130, 241–42n
oxytocin, 74, 82, 184–85, 217

Index

P

pain, 128, 141, 149, 157
  back, 63–64, 65, 97
  chronic, 96
  mindfulness and, 162
  social, 130, 223
painful emotions, 157, 198
panic attacks, 70–71, 202
parenting, 115, 121–22, 143–45, 204–25
  and amplifying good feelings, 213–15
  apologizing and, 211–12
  closeness in, and later disease, 114–15
  and confusing chronic unpredictable
    toxic stress with childhood
    challenges that foster resilience,
    207–9
  eye gaze in, 210–11
  hugs in, 217
  and instilling the four S's, 210
  intergenerational trauma and, 145,
    219–20
  and managing baggage, 207
  and managing reactivity, 206, 207
  and naming difficult emotions, 216–17
  by people with adverse childhood
    experiences, 115–21
  reliable adults or mentors and, 220–23
  school and, 223–25
  "Stop, Look, Go" method in, 215–16
  of teenagers, 121
  and validating and normalizing child's
    emotions, 212–13
  "what's happening" conversations in,
    217–19
past, 83–88
  reframing, 82
  see also memory(ies)
pediatric medicine, 232–33
pendulation, 189–90
Pennebaker, James, 158
physicians, 152–53, 229–31
pituitary-hypothalamus-adrenal stress axis,
  29–32, 76, 124, 211
placebo pills, 193
Pollak, Seth, 36–37, 246n
Porges, Stephen W., 210, 263n
Post Childhood Adversity Syndrome, 150
post-traumatic stress disorder (PTSD),
  xviii, 131, 137, 197, 199, 233
poverty, xviii, 233
prefrontal cortex, 49, 53, 105–7, 108, 211

pregnancy, 31, 101, 124
presidents, 62
primary biliary cirrhosis, 100
probiotics, 182
professional help, 160, 186–203
  Eye Movement Desensitization and
    Reprocessing, 198–201
  guided imagery, creative visualization,
    and hypnosis, 193, 194–96
  neurofeedback, 197–98
  Somatic Experiencing, 188–92
  therapy, 153, 186–88, 195
psoas, 178
psoriasis, 41, 183
psychotherapy, 153, 186–88, 195
  Eye Movement Desensitization and
    Reprocessing and, 198–201
PTSD (post-traumatic stress disorder),
  xviii, 131, 137, 197, 199, 233
puberty and adolescence, 102, 103, 107, 130
  brain and, 52–54
  see also teenagers

Q

qigong, 169

R

Race to Nowhere, 132
Rains, Mark, 257n
Raison, Charles, 172
Rashomon, 83
Reiki, 180
relationships, 143–46, 161
  brain and, 136, 137, 142, 145–46
  connecting and, 184–85
  Georgia and, 79
  good vs. bad interactions in, 214
  John and, 7, 134–36, 143
  Kat and, 142–43, 167
  unhealthy, entering or staying in, 139
reliable adults, 71–72, 74, 220–23
REM sleep, 199, 200, 201
resilience, 60, 65–66, 74–75, 81, 151, 172,
  224
  childhood challenges that foster, xvii,
    207–9
  reliable adult and, 71–72
  wobble and, 60–61, 63, 65–66
resilience score, 154–57
Ressler, Kerry, 110–11
rheumatoid arthritis, 98, 99

Rosenthal, Michele, 32–34, 46, 194–97
  alertness of, 39, 40
  hypnosis and, 194–96
rule-braking, 213

S
SAFE, 130
safe, in four S's, 210
Salzberg, Sharon, 169
Sapolsky, Robert, 31, 115
Schiller, Daniela, 198, 261n
schizophrenia, 48, 51, 124
school, 129, 131–34
  mindfulness in, 223–25
  stress from, 132–34, 223–24
  tests in, 133, 134, 224
secrets, 67–68, 71, 151, 217
secure, in four S's, 210
seen, in four S's, 210
Seery, Mark D., 63–66, 74
self, sense of, 137–38, 142, 228
self-awareness, 171
sensitivity hypothesis, 75 78, 80 81
serotonin, 75–76, 182, 183, 251n
sexual abuse, 11, 25, 31, 74, 108, 111,
    241–42n
  incest, 104
shame, 25, 68, 70, 141, 151
Shapiro, Francine, 198–203
shiatsu massage, 180
Shonkoff, Jack, 66, 72, 220, 232
siblings, 129
  loss of, 31
Siegel, Bernie, 157–58, 160, 179–80,
    192–93, 221, 228
Siegel, Dan, 52–53, 54, 138, 163, 170–72,
    204–5, 207, 208, 210, 211, 212,
    216, 221
Silver, Margery, 60
Sjögren's syndrome, 99, 100, 102
sleep:
  brain wash in, 262n
  REM, 199, 200, 201
smoking, 15
social engagement behaviors, 210
social pain, 130, 223
Solomon, Andrew, 227–28
Somatic Experiencing (SE), 188–92
Somatic Experiencing Trauma Institute, 189
soothing, 213
  in four S's, 210

Sotomayor, Sonia, 62
Steindl-Rast, David, 215–16
Stephen, 54–56, 109–10
  asthma of, 55
Stevens, Jane, 157, 225, 233–34, 257n
Stevens-Johnson syndrome (SJS), 33
stomachaches, 128
"Stop, Look, Go" method, 215–16
stress, 15, 16, 38, 65, 161
  adult support and, 72, 74
  brain and, 28, 29, 35–36, 122–23
  in children, damaging nature of,
    31–32
  chronic, 30–31, 37, 133
  chronic unpredictable, 41–43, 50–52,
    57, 60, 66, 122–23, 138, 153
  chronic unpredictable toxic, *see*
    Chronic Unpredictable Toxic Stress
  downshifted response to, 30
  empathic, 125
  genetics and, 75–78
  inflammation and, 29–32
  mindfulness based reduction of, 161,
    162, 168, 169, 224
  moderate, 66
  normative, 66
  of parents, children's absorbing of,
    124–27
  of parents, children's physical health
    and, 127–28
  perception of, 81–82
  predictable, 42
  rebounding from, 140
  reversing damage of, 58–59
  school, 132–34, 223–24
  in teens, 132–34
  in women vs. men, 103
stress axis, hypothalamus-pituitary-
    adrenal, 29–32, 37, 38, 76, 124, 211
stress hormones, xv, 30, 31, 36–38, 42, 66,
    76, 161, 162
  cortisol, 29, 30, 36, 38, 46, 77,
    100–101, 112, 124, 133, 161
Stress in America, 132
stress response, 35–37, 46, 185, 211, 246n
  fight-or-flight, 29, 36, 87, 101, 105, 128,
    138, 178
  as helpful, 82
  resetting, 151
  sensitivity gene and, 76
  toxic, 66–67

stroke, 16, 32
substance abuse, *see* addiction
suicide, 48, 157
Suomi, Stephen, 251n
synaptic connections, 24, 51, 52, 57, 84,
    142, 151, 171, 172, 206

T
tai chi, 169–70
Tartt, Donna, 145
teenagers:
    parenting of, 121
    and pressure to perform, 132
    stress in, 132–34
    see also puberty and adolescence
telomeres, 16
testosterone, 103
tests, 133, 134, 224
Theory of Desirable Difficulty, 62
Theory of Everything, 24–25, 58, 229
Therapeutic Touch, 180
therapy, 153, 186–88, 195
    Eye Movement Desensitization and
        Reprocessing and, 198–201
thyroiditis, 94, 98, 100
Tolstoy, Leo, 28
Tough, Paul, 208
toxic epidermal necrolysis syndrome
    (TENS), 33
toxic stress, chronic unpredictable, *see*
    Chronic Unpredictable Toxic
    Stress
toxic stress response, 66–67
Trauma Release Exercises (TRE), 178–79

U
ulcers, 32, 37, 42, 114
University of California, Los Angeles
    (UCLA), 182
University of California, San Francisco
    (UCSF), 16, 125–26
University of Cambridge, 25–26
University of Haifa, 124–25
University of Minnesota, 143
University of Rochester, 262n
University of Western Ontario, 137, 197

University of Wisconsin, 36
U.N. Rights of the Child, 233

V
vagus nerve, 210–11
van der Kolk, Bessel, 103–4
violence, xviii, 25, 31, 72, 233
vipassana meditation, 164, 166, 168, 169
visualization, 192–94, 195
vitiligo, 44, 45, 179
Vulnerability Hypothesis, 77–78, 80

W
Warner, Priscilla, 69–71
    EMDR therapy and, 202
    panic attacks of, 70–71, 202
Washington Post, 18
Waters, Sara, 125–27
Werner, Emmy, 257n
Whitaker, Robert, 225
Williamson, David, 242n
Wisconsin Study of Families and Work,
    104
wobble, 60–61, 63, 65–66
women, 89–113
    ACE Scores in, 104
    anxiety in, 96, 104, 107
    autoimmune disease in, 96–104,
        112–13
    childhood adversity in, 96
    chronic and ill-defined health problems
        in, 96–97, 103
    depression in, 48, 96, 97, 104, 107,
        110–13
    physiological differences between men
        and, 100
    stress and, 103
    and vulnerability of girls' brains,
        104–9
World Health Organization, 16, 56, 203,
    241n
writing, 157–60

Y
Yale School of Medicine, 36, 108
yoga, 177–78, 179

ABOUT THE AUTHOR

Donna Jackson Nakazawa is a science journalist and author of *The Last Best Cure*, the award-winning *The Autoimmune Epidemic*, and *Does Anybody Else Look Like Me?* as well as a contributor to the Andrew Weil Integrative Medicine Library book *Integrative Gastroenterology*. She has contributed to the *Washington Post, More, Glamour, Ladies Home Journal, Working Mother,* and *AARP the Magazine* as well as to blogs for *Psychology Today.* She is a graduate of Duke University and a recipient of fellowships from the Virginia Center for the Creative Arts, the MacDowell Colony, and Yaddo. She lives with her family in Maryland.